# THE
# BAREFOOT
# HOMOEOPATH

## Health Care
## for
## the Whole Person

Hyden House

615.532 HAR

Typeset, designed and published by
Hyden House Limited
Little Hyden Lane
Clanfield
Hampshire PO8 0RU
Great Britain
Tel: 0705 596500
Fax: 0705 595834


© 1991 Madeleine Harland and Glen Finn


Cover design by
Tim Harland, Hyden House Limited


Printed by
Biddles Limited, Guildford, Surrey


British Library Cataloguing in Publication Data
Harland, Madeleine, 1958-
    The barefoot homoeopath : health care for the
    whole person.
    I. Title II. Finn, Glen, 1953-
    615.532
    ISBN 1 85623 001 5

# THE AUTHORS

Glen Finn DHom, MHMA is a professional homoeopath with over ten years experience in practice. He has run many successful clinics in Britain, including a natural health centre. He has an excellent working knowledge of both chronic and acute prescribing and has taught homoeopathic courses to the general public for many years. Glen is a member of the Homoeopathic Medical Association. His wife, Elizabeth, is also a homoeopath.

Madeleine Harland BA, DipTHP, MCRAH has studied and used homoeopathy personally for the last ten years. She studied at the National School of Advanced Hypnosis and Psychotherapy and is a member of the Central Register of Advanced Hypnotherapists. Madeleine is also a qualified yoga teacher.

Glen and Madeleine are also authors of *Healthy Business - The Natural Practitioner's Guide to Success.* They lecture extensively throughout the UK to students and graduates of the natural medical professions and write for many general and specialised publications.

# CONTENTS

**SECTION TWO**
**Prescribing**
**The Art of Barefoot Homoeopathy**

# DEDICATION

To Liz and Tim who made this book possible.

# FOREWORD

by
Dr. Trevor M. Cook

The increasing popularity of homoeopathy and other natural therapies in recent years has led to a demand for more knowledge and for treatment that far exceeds the information services and qualified practitioners available. There is, therefore, a continuing need for more information and simple instruction that will enable lay people to treat themselves and their families for a variety of common, day to day ailments. This book is, therefore, a welcome addition to the help available.

Through this book, Madeleine Harland and Glen Finn aim to open up the world of homoeopathy and natural cures to make them accessible to everyone who wishes to use them. Rightly, they stress that homoeopathy is neither a cure-all nor an elixir of life, particularly with first aid and self care, but it is a safe, inexpensive and effective treatment for many common conditions if properly applied. The need for qualified medical attention for more serious conditions or those that do not respond to treatment is also stressed.

The format of the book is very straightforward and logical; from simple 'jargon free' explanations through actual treatments to useful information, including a Directory of Services. A unique feature is the inclusion of guidance on case management, diet, exercise, work and play.

I am sure this valuable book will enjoy the success it deserves.

*Trevor M Cook*

Dr. Trevor M. Cook
President, The United Kingdom Homoeopathic Medical Association
Principal, The Hahnemann College of Homoeopathy

# INTRODUCTION

## How This Book Works

*The Barefoot Homoeopath* is compiled and laid out in a way that is simple and easy to use, but still follows basic homoeopathic principles. Its purpose is to give you a comprehensive foundation of information which will enable you to tackle any common or minor health problem.

We begin at Section One with Chapter 1, explaining the 'barefoot' philosophy of personal first aid, preventative and self help health care. Chapter 2 discusses why homoeopathy can be successfully used as a primary measure in taking control of your own health. Chapter 3 looks at the history of homoeopathy, its origins and its place in our world. Chapter 4 explains how homoeopathy works and the processes involved in creating the remedies and their different potencies.

Chapters 5 and 6 then explore the idea of a practical holistic lifestyle. We examine how the 'barefoot' philosophy of self-empowerment can be extended to all aspects of your life and help you to find a more healthy, happy and balanced integration of mind, body and spirit. To find an inner harmony is no easy task, but it is the essence of true preventative medicine and holistic health care.

Section Two is the main part of *The Barefoot Homoeopath*, dealing with prescribing. Firstly, we explain such practical points as the storage of homoeopathic medication and how to select the right remedy in Chapter 7. Then, from Chapter 8 through to Chapter 17, we progress through the body starting with the head working downwards through to the chest, stomach, abdomen and the reproductive organs. We work our way outwards from minor backache and skin problems to common infectious diseases and simple first aid for stings, bites and bruises. Each chapter deals with a particular section of the body and the treatment of ailments relating to that section. Working through the body in this sequence allows us to follow basic homoeopathic laws (which will be explained later) described by the famous homoeopath, Constantine Herring:

*From above to below*
*From within to without*
*From the centre to the circumference*
*From major organs to minor organs*
*Symptoms disappear in the reverse order of their appearance.*

In Chapters 8 to 17 each health problem is listed with the relevant homoeopathic remedies (laid out in alphabetical order) and a description of the corresponding specific symptoms. This allows each remedy to be matched to the unwell individual. There is also a comprehensive index at the back of the book to help you find your way around with ease.

Because this book is specifically about common, but minor, ailments the list of homoeopathic remedies is restricted to the most frequently used medicines (there are over two thousand homoeopathic remedies available) and the ones found most generally effective for each problem.

Experience and practice over years has been our guide. We do strongly recommend that should you be worried about **any** symptoms or illnesses in yourself or another, however trivial, you should consult your G.P. for a diagnosis or a reputable, qualified natural medicine practitioner for treatment.

Finally, Chapter 18 concludes Section Two by offering guidelines on when to seek medical advice. Obviously, we cannot include every eventuality but the rule of thumb should be one of common sense.

At the end of the book we have included three appendices. Appendix 1 is a mini *materia medica* of remedies which lists all the homoeopathic remedies used in the book and the symptoms which would be most characteristically associated with each remedy. When prescribing from Section Two of the book, this *materia medica* can act as a useful cross-reference to ensure the selection of the right remedy. Appendix 2 is a directory of products and services and Appendix 3 is a recommended reading list. We hope you will find these sections of the book useful.

Homoeopathy has sometimes been veiled even from natural medicine enthusiasts by archaic language, apparently mysterious processes and a complex system of selecting remedies. Although the subtle and learned expertise of professional homoeopaths is never in question here, we feel that it is time that the use of homoeopathic medicines for simple illnesses and complaints becomes a straightforward choice for everyone. Simplicity is therefore the underlying principle in this book. We hope that you enjoy using it.

# SECTION ONE

Homoeopathy
and
the Barefoot Philosophy

# Chapter 1

# BAREFOOT HOMOEOPATHY EXPLAINED

As we progress technologically, many miracles have taken place in the realms of health care. Diseases which would have taken lives even ten years ago have become treatable. Intricate techniques in surgery can now offer hope and new life to thousands of patients. Additionally, for a few pence, many of the common 'third world' diseases like salt treatment for severe dehydration caused by diarrhoea, and vaccinations for cholera and hepatitis, have saved many thousands of lives. These are the show case stories, the pluses in the system.

The minuses also exist. Some of these are the serious side effects of certain drugs, escalating costs in the treatment of many diseases, shortages of hospital beds and essential equipment, and the fact that cures for many serious illnesses still elude scientists despite lucrative research programmes. Recent research also shows that many 'first world' countries suffer from an array of 'civilised' diseases which are apparently self-inflicted. Our comparative affluence seems to fuel ill health rather than prevent it. We exchange malnutrition and dysentery, for example, for heart disease and lung and bowel cancer.

As a consequence of these factors, many people turn to natural medicine because orthodox systems of health care have failed them. They often turn to natural medicine in desperation and as a last port of call. Even then, many find relief and some even a cure at the eleventh hour. But this is not the ideal. It would be far better for us to teach our children and ourselves simple natural methods of health care from a very young age and work on preventing illness and not only trying to cure it when it has taken hold.

This is the purpose of this book. We aim to chip away at health problems by offering a comprehensive system of first aid treatment and preventative health care. This is where the concept of 'barefoot' homoeopathy enters. The Chinese have a community self-help system which teaches preventative medicine and the treatment of first aid problems. They train health workers to deal with cuts and colds, health education (which includes information concerning the importance of adequate sewage disposal and clean water supplies), pre and post-natal care, contraception and the delivery of normal births. They also arrange for specialist medical care in serious cases. The appointed health carers often work part-time and continue with their jobs in the factory or the field. They are an integral part of the community and are called 'barefoot doctors'. Without mimicking the Chinese, we can take their idea and transform it for our own needs.

Our health systems in the West are complex and expensive. The initiative for finding solutions to the increasing problems of health care can, however, come from the individual. You do not need to be passive patients at all. Let every individual attend to the common and minor ailments and simple illnesses first and further prevent illness by common sense 'lifestyle management' as the first line of call. Let the professionals deal with the serious, life threatening diseases. It is, of course, a matter of choice as to whether you consult a natural medicine practitioner or a conventional doctor.

## Responsibility

Common problems like first aid and 'flu should come within the province of each individual's health care. Our health is our responsibility. The ability to use natural remedies with wisdom and judgement should rest with us. When all health concerns become solely the province of the professionals, we divorce ourselves from self-determination and personal responsibility. We are transformed into a somewhat anonymous patient who understands little of the workings of synthetic drugs and technical terminology. Common complaints call for simple solutions. Barefoot homoeopathy, with no side effects, can offer solutions to these problems. Let us then become 'barefoot' homoeopaths!

## Natural Skills

In this book we primarily cover all aspects of prescribing homoeopathy for simple health problems but we also include naturopathic tips, herbs and simple nutritional advice. To master these skills does not require a vast commitment of time or a huge pharmacy in your bathroom cupboard. It also does not require the adoption of any philosophical beliefs or a change in your style of clothes! All you need is a book which is clear and easy to refer to and a range of homoeopathic remedies which cover most common problems. Simple natural cures and tips are included in each section to give an additional arsenal in the quest for better health.

Most significantly, homoeopathic medicines, when given in low doses for simple problems, can never cause drug induced diseases or unpleasant side effects. The remedies can create reactions when taken in high potency or for a long period of time, but they cannot cause toxicity in the first aid situation. They are like computer software information; if they are not relevant (i.e. unnecessary or unrelated to the health problem), they are ignored and pass through the system. Additionally, the remedies can actually prevent uncomfortable complications such as persistent catarrh after a cold.

The aim of this book is to open up the fascinating world of homoeopathy and natural cures to make them accessible to everyone who wishes to use them. Just as many households reach for aspirin for headaches, more and more people are turning to homoeopathy to solve their health problems. There is no reason why we cannot prescribe these gentle but effective remedies in the home for a whole host of illnesses without the fear of side effects and complications.

By taking your health into your hands, you are not playing at doctors and nurses! Instead, you are empowering yourself and taking responsibility for your most precious asset, your quality of life. This empowerment is part of a whole spectrum of self-transformation which every individual has the right to explore. This book is the first in a series which will enable you to discover and effectively use a simple system of health care which is both a fascinating subject in itself and a powerful way of improving the lives of yourself, your family and friends.

# Chapter 2

# TAKING CONTROL OF YOUR HEALTH

Happily, homoeopathy is an increasingly popular form of natural medicine in the general public's mind. This is simply because it works! So many people have benefited from homoeopathic remedies that the power of the word of mouth has outweighed the scepticism of orthodox science which has yet to explain exactly **why** it works.

Not only does homoeopathy work well on adults, it also has a powerful healing effect on babies, children and animals and these cures are well documented. Babies and animals cannot be accused of having an illness that is 'all in the mind'. Therefore, homoeopathy's power cannot entirely lie in what is called the placebo effect. That is the power of suggestion carried by a blank pill. Patients believe that they are feeling better simply because a physician has given them a medicine. This is arguable and totally refutable in animals and very young children. Cows with mastitis care little whether their drinking water carries a remedy to heal their illness. They just drink. It is the farmer who knows by result that his homoeopathically treated cows are healthier and measurably less likely to suffer from mastitis.

## Drug Dependent Culture

Besides the ability of homoeopathy to treat a vast array of diseases, there is also the priceless benefit that homoeopathic remedies have no side effects. We live in a very drug dependent culture, both for our medicine and for our pleasure. We enjoy the stimulus of caffeine, alcohol, nicotine and chocolate in our daily lives. Many of us think little of taking prescribed drugs for minor ailments as well as for serious complaints. Doctors are frequently asked for antibiotics to treat colds and 'flu though they may have little or no therapeutic effect. In fact, antibiotics cannot distinguish between friendly and  unfriendly bacteria and kill off valuable microflora in the bowel which help to maintain the digestive harmony of the body. They also kill the friendly enzymes in the vagina and can cause thrush in women. Furthermore, the more we take antibiotics the less effective they become. Our body learns to resist them, so that ever stronger doses must be taken. Antibiotics can save lives. This is what they are for, not to treat minor complaints which do not respond well to them anyway.

Antibiotics are only one example of common prescribed drug abuse. We use pain killers to suppress the slightest ache and aspirin to suppress a hint of a fever. Homoeopaths and naturopaths argue that pain is a message that should be acknowledged and dealt with by natural remedies. A fever also has its purpose and should not be suppressed unless there is a real threat of fatality or fits. Fevers burn out the dross of disease and have a cleansing action on the body.

## Cocktails

We take tranquillisers habitually, sometimes mixing them with a cocktail of other drugs. We use antihistamines, cortisone and other steroids, inhalants, antidepressants, pick-me-ups, 'downers', blood thinners, diuretics... the pharmaceutical list is long. The side effects are rarely acknowledged unless they appear in the short term and are worse than the disease the drug treats. We have little idea of the long term effect of these chemicals in our systems over generations just as we were ignorant of DDT or CFCs until relatively recently. Our attitude to drugs is one of the consumer. We take them. They are convenient now and the consequences are for tomorrow.

The contraceptive pill is an example of a drug which has been on general release since the early 1960s. Yet we have no idea what the cumulative effects of this drug are over three or four generations of women. The daughters of the mothers who first took the pill are now mothers themselves and what of their children and their health and fertility? Scientific evidence has revealed that the pill effects the ability of women to conceive and can also be attributed to the rise in cancer of the breast and cervix, migraine, allergies, candida (thrush), vascular disease and poor mental health.

Who can research the endless combinations of drugs we take over a lifetime and understand and catalogue the outcome? It is a monumental task.

As the causes of our diseases also become apparently more subtle and obscure, the cures become more complex and expensive. Like a consuming nightmare we are forced to throw more and more money into the pot to find relief from AIDS, cancer, liver disease, kidney disease, coronaries, Alzheimer's, Parkinson's and so on.

The picture is in no way hopeless, however. The answer to this maze of treatment and disease is a more preventative approach and less toxic remedies. Firstly, we need to take our health into our own hands. It is accepted today that a sensible diet and regular exercise sets a child on the road to health. Habits acquired in childhood establish a strong basis for health in adulthood. Later on, moderation in alcohol consumption, a healthy diet and continued exercise maintain good health.

Equally important to good 'life management' is the use of natural medicines for illnesses. Orthodox medicine has its place in our society for life threatening illness, accidents and, for example, the treatment of severe pain in terminal illness. We would never wish to undervalue the skills required to remove appendices, mend broken bones and relieve the terrible suffering caused by terminal cancer and other agonising conditions. What we take issue with is the almost addictive passion for drug use for most ailments which can be treated naturally, especially if they are attended to before they become too chronic and debilitating.

### Acute & Chronic - What Do We Mean?

It is at this point that we need to define the terms 'acute' and 'chronic'. When an illness is acute, this means that the symptoms generally appear quickly. Common ailments such as colds, chicken pox, stings and sprains are acute ailments. So too, however, are the more serious and life threatening illnesses like meningitis and typhoid. Chronic ailments are long standing illnesses both serious and minor. For example, haemorrhoids, dandruff or persistent catarrh could be considered minor chronic complaints. Examples of serious chronic complaints are arthritis, psoriasis and ulcerative colitis. This book is specifically written to help in prescribing for **minor** ailments, both chronic and acute. The more serious and life threatening illnesses, again both acute and chronic, obviously require professional attention. If you have any doubts regarding the seriousness of a complaint, please consult Chapter 18.

Acute prescribing is usually carried out at home after accidents and for the common infectious diseases to which we are prone. Acute prescribing is useful in three situations. Firstly, when the illness or accidental injury like a sting, sprain, bruise or cut is not sufficiently serious to require qualified medical attention.

Secondly, to treat an illness or an accidental injury before you see your medical practitioner, but we do counsel caution in all instances of accident or injury. Besides learning how to prescribe homoeopathic medicines, we advise that you take a first aid course. Even the basics can prevent serious paralysis or even save a life.

The third instance when acute prescribing is invaluable is for infectious diseases such as 'flu or measles. The orthodox profession can do little but advise rest and doses of drugs like paracetamol, whereas homoeopathy can help speed the progress of the disease, hasten recovery and prevent lingering side effects.

Prescribing for chronic conditions is useful for problems like warts, rashes and menstrual complaints. Again, if these disorders become serious, it is essential to consult a qualified practitioner.

One of the most worrying problems to confront is a sick baby. Most mothers have little choice when faced with a teething or feverish child and tend to turn to paracetamol each time. There are occasions when infant's paracetamol may be necessary, such as when a child has a high fever and does not respond to the homoeopath's remedies. Paracetamol may offer the child (and the parents!) a few hours of rest and relief. It is not good, however, to turn to it habitually as it is a sedative and does affect the nervous system. It can also damage the liver when the prescribed dose is exceeded. There are many homoeopathic remedies which offer an alternative to paracetamol and do no damage to the young child.

In the same way there is a case for orthodox treatment in matters of life and death but not as a habitual stand-by. Additionally, as there is often no orthodox treatment available for illnesses such as 'flu and glandular fever and homoeopathy can offer so much relief, it seems practical then for us to learn this system and take responsibility for family health. If we only see our doctor when we really need to we would ease the burden on our health service.

## Orthodox and Alternative Medicine
## - Where They Belong

Unfortunately, there is too much polarised opinion between the extremist alternative fans and the utterly orthodox. There is a middle way through. Medical problems like broken limbs, septic appendices, meningitis, congenital heart malformations and terrible injuries caused by accidents obviously need orthodox medical attention. Other less severe complaints would be well served by natural medicine. We do not need aspirins for headaches and the long term use of tranquillisers for stress and tension. We should only ever use steroids as the last resort, not the first. Equally, the continual use of Ventolin for asthma and hypertensive drugs in overweight patients does not make good sense when there are more benign alternatives available.

On the other hand, homoeopathy is not a magical cure-all or an elixir of life. Instead, it is a holistic form of medicine which takes into account the mental, emotional and physical aspects of each individual and their surroundings. It is also a safe, inexpensive and effective way of treating simple illnesses and complaints that we all encounter in our daily lives. Homoeopathy does not look to the past and deny the value of scientific discoveries. It simply questions the habitual abuse of pharmaceutical products which are sold to us commercially. Homoeopathy offers all of us the opportunity to take charge of our own minor ailments effectively and take responsibility for our heaith. It opens up the world of natural medicine and its practical application in our lives and creates an opportunity for us to study a fascinating philosophy of medicine which was developed by a brilliant doctor, Samuel Hahnemann, in the eighteenth century.

# Chapter 3

# THE DISCOVERY OF HOMOEOPATHY

In the late eighteenth century, a German physicist called Samuel Hahnemann developed the theory and practice of homoeopathic medicine. Samuel Hahnemann was an outstanding man with a great mind who was born before his time. He was horrified by the medical practices in vogue in his day. These included blood letting and the use of unproven and faddy cocktails of substances created by apothecaries. These apothecaries were paid according to how many ingredients they included in their medicines and not in relation to how effective these potions actually were. Many of these late eighteenth century practices actually did more harm to the patient than good.

At the time of Hahnemann's transition from the orthodox or allopathic treatment of disease to the homoeopathic principle of cure, he was greatly ridiculed by his contemporaries and often persecuted. He became an outcast in his profession because he challenged the *status quo* of late 18th century medicine. He was consequently driven from one town to another, constantly harried and under pressure to feed his family. Material difficulties and professional adversity did not deter him, however. Not only was he a translator of many learned texts and a pioneer in medical reform, he also discovered and developed the homoeopathic system of medicine. Eventually, he was accepted into the faculty of the University of Leipzig where he began further research and teaching of homoeopathic principles and practice.

At Leipzig, he developed his revolutionary system of medicine and the study and use of homoeopathic principles gradually became more and more widely accepted across the world. Now homoeopathy is practised in many countries and known about throughout the world. In Great Britain there is a great tradition of successful homoeopaths. We have many doctors practising homoeopathy as part of their general practice and a number of homoeopathic hospitals. There are also many professional homoeopaths working outside the National Health Service, offering a valuable service to the general public. Homoeopathic remedies are also freely available by post or from chemists and health food shops, enabling everyone to treat simple complaints in the home without having to consult a professional.

## Healing Power

Homoeopathy, like so many of our words, is derived from the Greek words *homoios* and *pathos* and means 'like suffering' when translated. Homoeopathy is simply the medical practice of treating like with like. This principle was well known by the 5th century Greek, Hippocrates, and the great 16th century Swiss alchemist, Paracelsus. They recognised that there is a relationship between how medicinal substances or remedies can create disease in healthy people and how the same remedies can be curative for the sick. Samuel Hahnemann was well educated in classical philosophy and medicine and was a prodigious scholar. He came across these homoeopathic principles in the course of his work but his development of homoeopathic medicine was more from laboriously collecting and sifting information and experimentation than from culling the wisdom of writers through the ages.

Hahnemann's medical discoveries stemmed from the belief that human beings have a natural capacity to heal themselves and that the body constantly attempts to restore harmony. Symptoms, which are expressed when an individual is ill, are the body's way of overcoming disease or disharmony in a person and are not the disease itself. The physician's role is to discover the cause of the disease and to stimulate the body's ability to overcome it, thereby healing itself. It is not to suppress those symptoms and thereby merely cosmetically remove the appearance of the disease.

## The Vital Force - A Unique Orchestrated Intelligence

Hahnemann called the natural ability of the body to heal, the 'vital force'. From the moment of our conception, an intelligent source of energy comes into play to orchestrate the formation of the human body. From birth, and through our subsequent life, this uniquely orchestrated intelligence continues to restore and renew us, maintaining harmony and therefore health.

The vital force can be described as a river of energy which flows through us, constantly revitalising our physical selves. When this flow of energy is weakened and the vitality is depleted by, for instance, a physical injury, prolonged exhaustion and stress, long term unhappiness or an inherited weakness, the harmonious flow is disrupted and the body is unable to function as it should. This is like a hiccup or a record that becomes stuck on one particular note or a word of a song. We see this clearly expressed in patients whose attention is focused entirely on their physical and mental symptoms who talk constantly of their ills.

Symptoms are an expression of the vital force being disrupted and the body's attempt to adjust and overcome this disruption. They are a warning of disharmony. They should never consequently be suppressed and swept under the carpet by drugs. Current medical opinion still believes that symptoms are caused by the illness.  Homoeopathy, by contrast, sees symptoms as the body's reaction against the illness. The body is constantly seeking to establish and maintain harmony or good health. It attempts to overcome 'dis-ease' by creating outward symptoms. Homoeopathy seeks to stimulate and not suppress this reaction and thereby re-establish harmony and a cure.

If our basic constitution is strong, the vital force can cope with minor problems like a cut or a mild upset stomach and restore the physical balance quite naturally. When the constitution of a person is weak, the vitality has to constantly battle to maintain health. Consider the strains of today. They are different to yesterday's smallpox, diphtheria and typhoid in the West. Now, we battle with the side effects of drugs like steroids and antibiotics, industrial and agricultural pollution, and phenomena like 'executive stress'.

None of our medical systems can actually cure disease. It is nature working like a river of life that moulds and builds up organisms to struggle against and overcome disease. Medicines and techniques which are 'natural', work with nature and stimulate the healing ability of the body. They are like good compost for plants. Compost alone cannot take over nature's role and force the blueprint in each seed to grow and achieve its potential but it can make germination and growth more healthy and fruitful. In the same way, natural medicine encourages and enables the body to overcome disharmony or dis-ease by stimulating the inherent healing resources.

How healing 'works' is ultimately a mystery. Homoeopaths talk of the vital force, hypnotherapists call on the infinite ability of the subconscious mind, acupuncturists call this force Chi or Ki. Whatever discipline we use in the field of natural medicine, we are encountering an underlying thread which passes through them all, linking us to a potent and regenerative force which heals and restores harmony not only to the body, but potentially to the emotions, mind and spirit.

## Provings

Hahnemann's primary aim was to find a system of medicine which worked with the vital force and not against it. He began by studying various remedies which displayed this homoeopathic principle of like curing like. He was so convinced by his theories that he began by systematically testing them out on himself. He then worked with other healthy individuals. These tests were called 'provings'. They took various small doses of reputedly poisonous or medicinal substances over a long period of time, carefully documenting all the mental, emotional and physical symptoms they produced. Patients suffering from similar symptoms were then given the same substance that created these symptoms in the healthy individual. This gave very good results.

His painstaking research revealed undeniable evidence that the remedies not only created symptoms in the well but had curative powers on the sick. A simple example of this principle of *similia similibus curentur* (like cures like) is, for example, found in onions. It is well known that onions irritate the eyes and nose, whilst the homoeopathic remedy *Allium Cepa* (potentised onion) alleviates many of these symptoms which are found in the common cold. Another example is the honey bee which, when taken as the homoeopathic remedy *Apis Mellifica*, treats agonising stinging pains and red, blistered weals very effectively. An analogy of 'like cures like' is the practice of 'hair of the dog'. The substance, alcohol, which creates the hangover can alleviate the symptoms the next day - though we do not recommend this as a curative process!

Hahnemann's investigations led him to discover a number of guiding principles besides that of like cures like. These include how to select the correct remedy and how much of that substance should be given to the patient.

## The Infinitesimal Dose

The 'infinitesimal dose' has become the most characteristic feature of homoeopathy in the popular mind, although the word homoeopathy itself in no way includes infinitesimal in its meaning. The name homoeopathy only expresses its basic principle of similarity or like cures like. The infinitesimal dose is, however, as fundamental to homoeopathy as the law of similarity.

As we have already explained, Hahnemann discovered that substances which are poisonous in their natural state can be used to cure, but they can only cure diseases whose symptoms mirror or mimic the symptoms that are caused by the material dose. Another example of this process can be found in *Belladonna*, deadly nightshade. In its material state the berries are deadly, but in the form of a homoeopathic remedy, it treats many conditions including high fevers, delirium, scarlet fever-like sore throats, menopausal flushing, mastitis and boils.

Hahnemann began by giving himself and his followers material doses of substances like quinine, the malarial medicine, which produces fevers, sweating, flushing and rigours when given to a healthy individual but cures those symptoms when given to someone who has malarial symptoms. He quickly realised that many medicinal substances are very poisonous in their material state and that they could not be proved without very unpleasant side effects. He therefore began to dilute substances, such as arsenic and deadly nightshade, to avoid these side effects.

As Hahnemann systematically proved many remedies, he developed a special system of dilution which he later called 'potentisation'. He found that the more a similar remedy was diluted, the more effective it became. He also found that if he diluted substances in a strict sequence of ever increasing dilution, certain potencies or measured intervals of dilutions were more powerful than others. These serial dilutions were called 'potencies' to indicate the power of each interval. (Homoeopathic potencies will be fully explained in the next chapter.)

The use of minute doses is a necessary corollary of the principle of like curing like. The great power of the infinitely little and the opposite effect of large doses of substances has been demonstrated in nutritional research. For example, vitamins and minute traces of certain minerals are necessary in maintaining well-being in body and mind. In large doses, many are extremely toxic and, in some cases, they can actually create disease.

But how can a remedy which produces the symptoms of a disease be also the instrument of its cure? The reason in part may be found in the opposite effect of large and small doses on cells in the body. These have been demonstrated by experiments with yeast and *Arsenicum Album* (potentised arsenic). Whilst large doses of the poison, arsenic, actually destroyed yeast cells, very small doses actually stimulated their growth.

Thus was demonstrated in a simple organism what Hahnemann had discovered in regard to the more complex organism of the human body. He had shown that by sub-division and dilution, a drug may be transformed into a very powerful agent which, when applied homoeopathically, can stimulate the body in its fight against disease.

While Hahnemann tested a large number of drugs on himself, other provings were made with the co-operation of several members of his family and enthusiastic followers of his new system. This process of proving has been going on ever since and provings of otherwise untried substances are still being made.

The provings of symptoms which these substances can cause when given to a healthy person have been systematically catalogued in a book known as a *materia medica*. There are several versions available, compiled by different homoeopaths, all essentially the same but varying in the depth of detail. As they are written in precise language with listings of mental, emotional and physical symptoms, the detailed descriptions of each remedy can be accurately matched with the symptoms described by patients.

In this book we provide a simple *materia medica* (page 153) of all the homoeopathic remedies we list for the treatment of common ailments and first aid situations. This acts both as a reference and as a way of becoming familiar with the homoeopathic remedies. The more familiar one is with the remedies, the more their characteristics come alive and the easier it is to remember their differing pictures.

## How Homoeopaths Prescribe

How do homoeopaths arrive at the correct remedy? They never forget that there is really no such thing as a disease in the abstract: there are only sick people. The whole individual is always in their minds. They realise that the whole person is more than the sum total of his or her organs and that it is better to treat the sick person rather than the disease. To do this, they need to find out many details about their patients. These include their past health; the circumstances in which they live; the pattern of health in the family; the present condition and aspects of the personality which make each patient a distinct individual. Are they happier in hot weather or cold? Do they like the seaside or the mountains? Are they dark, red or fair haired? Does the patient fear thunder? Do they prefer to be alone or in company and when taken ill, does he or she want to be made a fuss of or to be left severely alone? Are they sulky or easy going? Are there any distinct food cravings? What are the hopes, fears and aspirations of each individual?

It is through such observations and understanding that the patient's whole personality becomes a guide to the homoeopathic remedy. All these questions enable the homoeopath to build up a multi-dimensional picture of the patient which will be matched to one of the drug pictures derived from the provings of remedies in the *materia medica*.

## Holistic Philosophy & Barefoot Homoeopathy

Selecting a homoeopathic remedy for a first aid situation or for a simple complaint requires less involved and lengthy research into a patient's individuality than a homoeopath would undertake for a more serious ailment. There is still, however, a relationship between how the person reacts to the illness and the individual remedy. For example, one person with 'flu may suffer most from aching limbs and chilliness. Another may suffer most from a fever with an upset tummy. Another, a sore throat and a congested chest. All could be diagnosed as suffering from 'flu, but they would each require different homoeopathic remedies. No single homoeopathic remedy for 'flu will be appropriate for everyone.

This process is, in fact, very simple, especially when we wean ourselves off the 'philosophy' of conventional medicine which usually offers us only one or two drugs for a problem and merely treats the symptom and not the person (i.e. headache = pain = painkiller = aspirin/paracetamol). In this way, simple first aid, or barefoot homoeopathy, still acts in a holistic manner as the remedy selected definitely fits **the individual**, even on the most simple level of two or three leading (i.e. most important) symptoms.

## Orthodox Science & Homoeopathic Philosophy

The concept of the infinitesimal dose has caused great scepticism and ridicule ever since it was developed. Scientists ask how a remedy which is only present in a sub-molecular dose can be effective. New discoveries have demonstrated that there are indeed peaks of energy at the specific dilution intervals of homoeopathic potencies. The changing outlook of science, coupled with highly sophisticated and finely calibrated space technology, is beginning to force a more open mind towards this mystery.

Because it is the individual that is treated and not the disease, the medical practice of running drug trials on disease states is problematic. Say, for instance, a trial is run on the use of *Rhus Tox* (poison ivy) for the treatment of arthritis and all patients being tested with homoeopathy are given *Rhus Tox* as their remedy. Using conventional double blind trials *Rhus Tox* cannot properly be judged as it does not suit all arthritis sufferers. This is because not all arthritis sufferers display the same symptoms which are appropriate for the use of *Rhus Tox*. Therefore, this kind of trial is unsuitable.

There have been other trials run to test homoeopathic medicines and some have acknowledged the need for the preselection of patients with symptoms which would require the same remedy. These trials are still, however, based on prescribing solely on the basis of the patients' set of symptoms which relate to a single diagnosed disease like, for example, seasonal rhinitis (hayfever). The efficacy of the remedy selected is then tested and compared to orthodox medication for the same disease. The trials do not allow the prescription of remedies for the whole person, taking into account his or her physical, emotional and mental details. This way of prescribing relies only on physical symptoms which is acceptable for minor problems but not for serious illnesses. Homoeopathy cannot be clinically tested and accurately judged in this way.

The moral of this tale is that one remedy for one diagnosed illness cannot be tested in orthodox clinical trials in the conventional manner. Homoeopathy must be tested according to homoeopathic principles, i.e. patients suffering from the same disease will often require different remedies. Also a number of different patients, all with differing health problems, may well benefit from the same remedy if their symptoms match the 'drug picture' appropriate for their remedy. Until scientists can grasp these fundamental principles, they will fail to give homoeopathy a fair trial.

# Chapter 4

# HOW HOMOEOPATHY WORKS

Homoeopathic remedies are made from substances found in the animal, vegetable and mineral kingdom and they are all given in a diluted, 'potentised' form. The honey bee, ants, snake venom and milk taken from a lactating dog, are some examples of 'animal' remedies which have great curative effects. The 'vegetable' remedies include herbs, botanical medicines and plants, their fruits, flowers, roots or berries. Also used are some plants which have no apparent medicinal effects in their natural state like club moss. From the 'mineral' kingdom substances like gold, calcium and phosphorus are used. Medicinal drugs like morphine and cocaine also find their place in the homoeopathic pharmacy. They are no longer poisonous, of course, because they are taken in an infinitesimal dose but, like all homoeopathic remedies, they are extremely effective when given to the right patient. Additionally, other substances which have little or no apparent curative effect on the human body in their natural form are also potentised and work as powerful remedies. These include common salt, sand, charcoal and pencil lead.

There are over two thousand homoeopathic remedies, each with their own 'drug picture', which has been painstakingly acquired by the detailed recording of provings. Many of these remedies have limited, very specific symptoms and are only used by practising homoeopaths for patients with serious illnesses. There are, however, a number of very commonly used remedies which treat many illnesses and minor complaints because they encompass a wide range of symptoms. These more commonly used remedies are called 'polychrests' and they are very effective when prescribed for acute or minor complaints as well as for the homoeopath's more serious cases.

## Mother Tinctures - The First Step

Creating a mother tincture is the first process in the manufacture of a homoeopathic remedy made from soluble substances. A material substance, like a plant, is taken and infused in up to 98% alcohol for up to three weeks. The resulting infusion is then strained through muslin and stored in a large jar. This liquid is called the 'mother' tincture and is represented by the symbol ∅. It is this mother tincture which is used in the first step of potentisation.

Mother tinctures can also be very useful for first aid when diluted with water and used externally, for example, on wounds or as an eye wash. They are rarely placed directly on the skin undiluted, except in the case of warts.

## Potencies Explained

There are a number of different scales of potencies. The two most commonly used scales are the 'centesimal' and 'decimal' scales.

## The Centesimal Scale

The most common potency available to the public is the 6c, generally labelled as '6', although 30c is sometimes available and is similarly labelled as '30'. The 'c' denotes the centesimal scale and originates from the Roman symbol for one hundred. It is not usually printed on the label in the United Kingdom but on the Continent the centesimal scale is written as 'CH'. If you are searching for *Arnica 6c* in Switzerland or France, it is easily identified by the label *Arnica 6CH*. In Britain, the number 6 will automatically mean the potency is in the centesimal scale.

To make a centesimal remedy, one part of the mother tincture is diluted with 99 equal parts of water/alcohol mixture and succussed (vibrated) for a few seconds. This will make a 1c potency. When one part of the 1c potency is then taken and diluted with a further 99 parts water/alcohol and again succussed, this makes a 2c potency. This process is then repeated a further four times to make the 6c potency and then a further twenty-four times, if required, to make the 30c potency. By the time a remedy becomes a 30c potency, it contains none of the original material substance and we are entering the realms of the sub-molecular!

## The Decimal Scale

The decimal scale is made in a similar manner with 'x' denoting this scale rather than 'c'. One part of the mother tincture is diluted with 9 parts water/alcohol and is succussed for a few seconds. Then one part of the 1x potency is then taken and added to 9 parts water/alcohol and succussed again. This process takes place a total of six times to create a 6x potency. In the decimal scale, homoeopaths generally use the 1x, 2x, 3x and 6x. The decimal scale is always denoted by an 'x' in Britain and by a 'D' on the Continent.

## Trituration - Processing Insoluble Substances

Insoluble minerals cannot be made into mother tinctures. To get over this problem and still achieve the accurate dilution of a substance, the mineral is diluted by adding one part of the mineral to 99 parts (or nine parts if the decimal scale is being used) of lactose powder and grinding them up with a pestle and mortar. This process is called 'trituration'. The dilution is then repeated, i.e. one part of the first mixture is added to a further 99 (or nine according to the scale used) equal parts of lactose and ground again. Dilution is repeated for a third time in exactly the same way. After this third trituration, the substance has reached a 3c (or 3x) potency. At this stage, it becomes dissolvable and can continue to be potentised in the usual manner in a dilution of water and alcohol.

Homoeopaths use a wide range of potencies according to the nature of the remedy and the patient in front of them. The most commonly used potencies are taken from the centesimal scale and are the 6, 30, 200, 500, 1000 (called M), 10,000 (10M), 50,000 (50M) and 100,000 (CM). Centesimal potencies from 200 upwards are only available to professional homoeopaths and they are prescribed with great care. Homoeopathy turns conventional pharmacy on its head. The higher the potency, the less there is of the original material substance. Yet the less the original substance there is, the more powerful its action.

The exact intervals of these potencies were discovered by homoeopaths over many years using meticulous experiments. Scientific invention has now caught up with practical application and it has been discovered that the energy inherent in the remedy peaks at these intervals. In other words, the remedies have a greater activity in these chosen potencies than in others like, for instance, 48c or 506c! It will not be long before quantum physics is capable of decoding these sub-atomic energy surges and gives us a clear answer to why the remedies work.

To avoid confusion, this book assumes that the reader will be using the 6c and 30c potencies for homoeopathic remedies. The most commonly used remedies, listed in this book, are generally available in these potencies from your local homoeopath, health food shops, some chemists or by post from specialist suppliers. (See Appendix 2 on page 181 for a directory of mail order suppliers.)

## Biochemic Tissue Salts

In 1873, a German doctor of medicine, Dr. W. H. Schuessler, began to publish a series of papers on the subject of body tissue salts. He had decided that homoeopathy was too complicated. He thought that there were too many remedies, each with a detailed picture of mental, emotional and physical symptoms, which made prescribing a lengthy and complex art. Dr. Schuessler claimed that all that was necessary to re-establish balance in the body were minute doses of the body's twelve essential body chemicals. These would act as a stimulus and rectify any imbalances. He therefore formulated the twelve biochemic tissue salts.

At first there was an outcry from classical homoeopaths who followed Hahnemann's methods to the letter. Eventually, homoeopaths acknowledged that the tissue salts did have a curative effect and that the simple system was indeed tailor-made for home prescribing. The tissue salts were recognised as an excellent first aid system. Today, many homoeopaths also use the salts in conjunction with constitutional homoeopathic prescribing and find them an effective and useful addition to conventional homoeopathy.

As the tissue salts are mainly derived from mineral (i.e. hard or insoluble) matter, they have to be made by the process of trituration. They are systematically diluted in a mortar with *sac lac* (lactose) powder and crushed with a pestle for a specified period of time. Biochemic tissue salts are also potentised to a sixth decimal scale (6x) although not in exactly the same way as homoeopathic remedies.

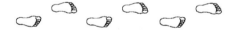

This chapter concludes our introduction to homoeopathy and the principles which underpin its practice. For barefoot homoeopaths, homoeopathy is not the only string to the self-help bow. There is also the additional dimension of lifestyle management and aspirations towards a more balanced and whole life. This balancing of the demands of work, play and family life is a challenging concern. To integrate the needs of mind, body, emotions and spirit and to find an inner harmony is no easy task, but it is the essence of true preventative medicine and holistic health care.

# Chapter 5

# HOLISTIC HEALTH CARE

Holistic health care is caring for the whole person and not just the physical body or even the mind. It takes into consideration the emotional fulfilment and happiness of every person, their intellectual potential, their personal beliefs and spiritual base. This chapter can only be a door opening on this large subject, but it is a beginning. None of us who are concerned with 'total health' can ignore the necessity for a holistic vision. Just as we should not patch up bodies whilst ignoring anguished minds, we have to acknowledge the relationships which exist between our bodies, emotions, minds, spiritual aspirations and, ultimately, our planet Earth. The deeper we go into ourselves, the more apparent are the subtle connections between our personal equilibrium and the health of our world. We cannot have a healthy body and a sick planet.

## Food

Many books and articles have been written about diet and health in the last two decades. A healthy diet, once thought of as food fit for rabbits and eccentrics, has now entered the province of common sense. There is now a wealth of information regarding a healthy diet and how to cook wholefoods in an appetising manner.

How we cook our food is very important. Today, very few people add bicarbonate of soda in the cooking process to make their vegetables more tender and green-looking because it destroys the vitamin content of the food. We also try not to boil our vegetables to death and many people now steam food instead. A further extension of enlightened cooking is to prepare food without using any water, fat or salt. To do this, you need 'waterless cookware' which has a special thermic base. It is hygienic, energy saving and can cook any type of food. Not only is it healthier than conventional cooked food, the flavour of the food prepared in waterless cookware has to be tasted to be believed!

Many people are now aware of the necessity of a healthy diet and research has proved what many naturopaths and homoeopaths have suspected for decades. We know that death from coronary heart disease is highest in countries (mainly the industrialised nations) which eat the largest proportion of animal foodstuffs, including meat and dairy products. Vegetable protein scores high in a healthy diet, it is radically less fattening, and some vegetable fibres can actually lower blood cholesterol.

Additionally, the high animal fat and cholesterol diet which causes heart disease also causes cancer of the colon, breast and uterus. This diet is low in fibre and high in cancer-causing agents. This is a dangerous combination. The carcinogenic substances sit in the gut for longer due to the lack of fibre and are reabsorbed into the system. They then wreak their havoc.

Vegetables like spinach, broccoli, the various cabbages, cauliflower, turnips and brussels sprouts also help the body to resist the development of cancers. We all produce mutated cells. Healthy bodies naturally reject them from the system. Evidence now shows that many cancers are not merely accidents of fate. Like smoking and lung cancer and the excessive consumption of alcohol and stomach and liver cancer, what we eat can directly affect the possibility of becoming prey to specific cancers.

Added to the dangers of disease, most of our animal products are produced in such an artificial and barbaric manner that it seems inconceivable that these foods are healthy. We force five battery hens into a cage 18 by 20 inches and crop their beaks so that they cannot kill or mutilate each other. The RSPCA would prosecute us if we treated our budgerigars in this fashion. We feed calves on diets low in iron and confine them in the dark so that the veal is white. We also make their stalls so tiny that they cannot turn around. This is to reduce the risk of damage and to keep their flesh tender.

We confine pigs and cows so that they do not build up 'unnecessary' muscles. We pump them full of hormones to stimulate growth and antibiotics to prevent disease, feed them offal made from their own kind and herd them into cramped trucks to send them to slaughter. They die agitated and terrified. There is a fundamental inconsistency at work when we make a mechanised factory out of a farm yet claim that we are a nation of animal lovers.

## Sustainable Agriculture

There are alternatives. We can grow vegetables ourselves, free from petro-chemical pesticides and fertilisers. Organic growing does not need to be complicated or difficult. Even if a person has no garden, food can be grown in a confined space in window boxes and on window sills or balconies. We know a couple who have a garden which is five foot by three foot. In this space they grow runner beans, tomatoes, strawberries, broccoli, and peas (and alfalfa and bean sprouts on their window sill all year round!).

Of course, it is easy to buy food from supermarkets and shops but there are important reasons why we should try to wean ourselves off this convenient habit. A few of these are as follows: the multitude of chemicals used in intensive agriculture are poisoning our environment and ultimately ourselves; intensive agriculture is also responsible for worldwide soil erosion, thereby depleting one of nature's greatest resources; the major cost in most foodstuffs is transportation (particularly when imported) and packaging which are both heavily dependent on non-renewable resources. This is a waste and a drain on the world's resources and the environment in general; ecological concerns aside, food grown organically in your own garden quite simply tastes far better!

New methods of producing food without destroying our world are being constantly evolved. An example is 'Permaculture', a sustainable, low maintenance, organic method of growing food and fuel crops which works in harmony with the features of the local environment and its wildlife. Furthermore, each person can grow what is suitable for their circumstances. We may not be able to start smallholdings in the country. We may live in the city with a small garden. But we can do something and make ourselves more intimate with the seasonal processes of sowing, germinating, growing and harvesting, even if it is only tomatoes in the window box and bean sprouts on the sill!

Growing plants is also an opportunity to take our interest in natural medicines into another sphere, by planting herbs with vegetables. Not only does this repel pests, it allows us to cultivate a variety of useful teas and medicines and to study plants which, when potentised into homoeopathic remedies, become powerful medicines. Growing them can become a fascinating hobby.

Farms producing meat from animals reared in free range circumstances, fed on food untainted by hormones and general 'herd' medication and killed in a more humane manner are also springing up. It is true that 'real' meat is more expensive than the pre-packed supermarket meat but it is worth 'going without' so you can have the occasional treat. At least you know what you are eating and it also tastes considerably better.

Not everyone wants to become a vegetarian, give up drinking alcohol entirely, take to the soil or eat an exclusively wholefood diet. This is a personal choice. But what we can be aware of is the value of moderation. Obviously, a diet which emphasises high fat, low fibre, too much alcohol, caffeine, sugar and carbohydrates is very negative. It creates physical ill health, including cancer, heart disease and obesity, and can cause emotional ill-health, mood swings and a general lack of vitality. It is not a harmonious and happy way of treating one's body. If you find yourself trapped in one or a combination of these habits, seek help.

We say little here about tobacco smoking. The evidence is clear. It is a horribly destructive habit, both to ourselves and the others who are forced to endure vicarious smoking.

Finally, what we eat and drink in childhood can have a far greater legacy than we imagine and can affect the habits of a lifetime. Research has demonstrated that there is a relationship with diet and addictions. Children raised on a diet full of stimulants like sugar and caffeine can often develop addictive tendencies in adulthood and have a greater than average tendency to abuse drugs, alcohol, tobacco or binge on food. Clearly, preventative health care must stem from balance and moderation, even in early life.

## Exercise

Like healthy diets, exercise has become very much in the public eye and a part of fashion. Whatever your preference, whether you choose low impact aerobics, yoga, golf or Tai Chi, enjoy yourself and exercise regularly. Like other aspects of health care, excessive habits and fanaticism are unhealthy. Do not become an exercise freak!

Remember also that walking at a moderate pace for an hour a day is the most natural, effective form of exercise and is equal to running for approximately half an hour four days a week. Brisk walking increases the heart rate, tones the muscles and decreases body fat. It is also gentle on the body. Walking is a good choice of exercise for those who are uncomfortable with competitive sports or who do not have time for gyms. Walking is also ideal for older people and for people recovering from a health problem. Needless to say, if you have been unwell, consult your practitioner before embarking on any new form of exercise.

Digging a vegetable patch can also kill two birds with one stone. 'Working out' outside can be hugely beneficial to personal fitness and to the larder. Being in the fresh air and living with the seasons can also give us a sense of deep personal richness. We become more aware of our local wildlife, of the ever-changing weather and of the miraculous way in which nature generates life and gives us food. It teaches us to appreciate rain and sun, the cycles of the year and gives us simple insights into ourselves and the planet which we share.

## Work

Most of us have to work for a living, whether it is caring for our families or earning a wage. Often it is both. Some form of work is an essential aspect of living a balanced life. Those that enjoy their work are very lucky, especially if their job has a holistic angle to it and is not merely concerned with paying the rent or mortgage. If a job is creative, has some kind of ethical drive behind it and actively considers the needs of people and the environment on a local if not global scale, it is bound to be far more fulfilling than just working for money. Wealth is ephemeral. Let us work for a world that is not.

Many people do not have the chance to work in so called 'alternative' careers but we all have choices that we can make about how we live. If we attempt to live and work with minimum harm to people and the planet and attempt to find a more sustainable, ecologically and socially friendly way of life - and it is possible! - then we will find that our psychological, as well as global, health will improve. Alienation stems quite simply from a lack of contact. Positive steps towards a more harmonious way of living is the way to overcome alienation.

## Play

Besides work, there must be play. There have to be areas of space in everyone's life and the time to unwind and relax. For some, a game of squash is just that. For others, sports are definitely not relaxing. Whatever your pleasure, whether it is mountain climbing, macrame, beekeeping or building models, devote time to it. You deserve some respite from life's busyness.

Like hobbies, holidays are equally important, even if you take the telephone off the hook and go out for the day. Holidays are a rest from routine. We all need that. We often try to live within our routines because we become afraid to step outside of them. If life is lived according to immutable rules, we stultify in the boredom and predictability of it. Everyone needs a change and a rest. If you cannot afford a trip abroad, visiting a friend who has moved out of the area could be a good plan. A change of air can create new perspectives and insights into our day to day lives and can be plain good fun.

## Inner Health

Besides sensible lifestyle management like a good diet, exercise, relaxing and taking holidays, there is also the question of emotional health. It is important to cultivate good relationships with other people. If we are at war with others, it usually indicates that we are at war with ourselves. Anger, inflexibility, selfishness, habitual worrying... these are qualities which create tension and disharmony. They can not be swept away with artificial goodwill. They have to be faced and understood. If your problems are apparently insurmountable, find a sympathetic ear, whether personal or professional. Try to understand what causes these negative responses.

Understanding ourselves usually comes with time. It is important to try and come to terms with our failings and general personality but not to delve so deeply into them that we become obsessed. There is nothing worse than the cliché of the psychologically self-obsessed individual who constantly analyses him or herself but is fundamentally well! Part of travelling the road towards self-acceptance and understanding is cultivating a conscience about our actions but not becoming over self-critical. We should genuinely attempt to interact harmoniously with our social environment and we should accept, without complacency, our shortcomings. This is a tall order but not impossible. Feeling guilty about ourselves can serve no purpose. It is the other side of being self-obsessed. We have to tear ourselves away from the habit of guilt and come to terms with its origins.

Many people regard the world as an inhospitable place in which individuals have to learn to cope. They feel alien and alone. Because life is a day to day battle at 'the front' of experience, many of the small but uplifting experiences are lost in the fray.

One of the secrets of happiness is to find pleasure and value in the apparently insignificant aspects of life. This is not to become trite or superficial but to recognise the worth in things like the new growth in spring or a kind gesture from someone in the street. Beneath this is the philosophy that the world is a fundamentally benign place and that the majority of people are basically kind and good. These beliefs are not necessarily religious but are part of many religions. Once adopted it is surprising how the prophecy fulfils itself. Negativity thrives on itself and so too does optimism and kindness. Every day we create the lives we live. Most of us who have the freedom to read, study and interact with others have the power to transform our lives. If this ability is tainted by pessimism and bitterness, we damage our own potential and contribute to a dismal negativity which helps no one.

## Dreams and Aspirations

Inner health needs inspiration. Being too insular, as if our life is lived in a sealed jar, is airless and stale. We all need to cultivate adventure, even if it is on our doorstep. We also need to meet new people and be introduced to new ideas. Learning should continue to the grave. We never lose our potential to grow.

Part of this process of change is the necessity of having dreams or aspirations. Call these 'goals' or whatever name you like. Another secret of happiness is the ability to make real one's dreams. To do this we have to work from where we are. Having exclusively impossible goals is as sad as having no dreams at all. If our goals are too big and are unrealistic, we will not succeed. We will become cynical and disenchanted with ourselves and the world. If they are too small, we sell ourselves short.

It is important to choose our goals carefully and take time to visualise them every day. Take a few moments regularly and mentally work towards achieving these ambitions. Work in a practical way towards realising these goals as well. Do not give up and do not underestimate the power of thought. The human being is a creature of extraordinary potential. What is necessary is to choose wisely what you really want.

Besides personal goals, do not give up giving to others either. Though we cannot mortgage ourselves to the pains of the world, we can still help other people, even if our role is seemingly trivial. Unhappiness and a sense of isolation often stems from being insular and out of contact with those around us. The best way to get back in touch is to reach out and give.

## Complementary Medicine

Finally, if you do develop a health problem, despite a healthy lifestyle, try to deal with it naturally as the first line of call. If it is outside the province of self-treatment, visit a reputable practitioner. Natural medicine works to restore harmony in the body and does not merely seek to suppress the symptoms. It is also effective in many different areas of treatment. Find out what various natural health disciplines are available in your area. Also check the qualifications and reputation of your potential practitioner. A good natural health practitioner is a very valuable friend.

If you require the services of conventional medicine, find out if you can use natural medicine in a complementary manner. For example, homoeopathic remedies can do much to assist the healing of broken bones and surgical wounds. A practitioner's advice on diet and dietary supplements can also aid recovery during illness and convalescence. Hypnotherapy techniques, counselling, Bach Flower remedies and certain homoeopathic remedies can offer relief from emotional trauma. These are a few examples of 'complementary' medicine. Orthodox practitioners are increasingly opening their minds and their doors to alternatives to conventional medicine because they are so effective.

# Chapter 6

# NATURAL CONCLUSIONS

Natural medicine as a whole is a marriage of ancient and modern. Practitioners of acupuncture and Chinese herbalism draw upon knowledge which is many thousands of years old. The medicinal qualities of plants used by medical herbalists are part of what was an esoteric or secret knowledge that has been passed down through the centuries in both the East and West. Many of the psychotherapy and counselling techniques used today are innovative, breaking new ground in our perception and understanding of ourselves. Other techniques such as hypnosis, visualisation and meditation used therapeutically for a far wider brief than just to relax and 'feel good', have origins which are also ancient.

It is true that homoeopathy was discovered and developed relatively recently in comparison to some disciplines like acupuncture and Ayurvedic medicine. Some of its roots, however, can be traced back to the ancient Greeks and the Swiss alchemist, Paracelsus, and its laws such as *similia similibus curentur* or 'like cures like' were familiar to Hippocrates. Much of the wisdom of the Greeks originated from the Egyptians and the Egyptians in turn acquired much of their knowledge from the ancient sages of the East. Wisdom is a universal tree and its fruits have spread through many civilisations and cultures. Although homoeopathy does have a relationship with ancient laws and principles, it is essentially a modern practice.

Homoeopathy has a subtle and profound power. Professional homoeopaths who prescribe remedies for serious and long-standing complaints describe how patients can literally regenerate during a course of treatment. This healing process occurs on many levels. For example, a patient who came for homoeopathic treatment for a skin complaint found that a long term ailment of intermittent sleeplessness, which he had not regarded as important enough to mention, had also cleared up. Another example is one of a patient who had never been well since contracting glandular fever five years before. Homoeopathy not only cleared up the physical symptoms of weakness, a sore throat and swollen glands but also relieved the patient of feelings of anxiety and depression which had lingered after the illness.

## Barefoot Healing

The curative power of homoeopathy is not just evident when professionals prescribe for chronic conditions. The 'barefoot' homoeopath can also witness positive transformations in the health of himself or herself and those around him or her. To illustrate this, we offer three examples of barefoot healing.

We have a friend who contracted a dose of chicken pox in her mid-thirties. Her temperature ran at 102 degrees for three days and besides being covered in itching, burning blisters, she had a terrible headache. Her G.P. advised rest and painkillers if her discomfort became too unbearable and left her to get on with it. Two remedies, *Rhus Tox* and *Pulsatilla*, were tried without any results. Then she was given *Apis Mellifica 30*, primarily for the violent, stabbing headache and then the burning fever. She began to recover within the hour and she was given two more doses. Her great discomfort was relieved within three hours. The chicken pox became a temporarily unsightly affliction but was bearable. (Incidentally, during the height of the fever, she was sponged with cool water to bring down her high temperature.) Her recovery was without any complications.

Our second example is one of a colleague with a broken bone. He broke his collar bone whilst practising a martial art. He was advised to take *Symphytum 6* (potentised comfrey) night and morning for a week and then a lesser frequency of once a day for a further two weeks. He also rubbed comfrey ointment into the area around the fracture. When he went back to the hospital for a check up after six weeks, the doctor commented that he had never seen a collar bone heal so quickly and cleanly.

Finally, another friend suffered from an uncomfortable skin complaint for many months. In the course of her job, she handled freshly baked bread and other foodstuffs every day. She consequently had to wash her hands frequently and they became dry, sore and developed painful, red, dirty looking fissures at the end of each fingertip. She took *Graphites* 6 night and morning for three weeks. During this time the condition completely cleared up and has never returned.

We could fill a book of stories about homoeopathy and how it has helped both humans and animals with simple, straightforward problems and more difficult, long-lasting illnesses. The message behind this is that homoeopathy is a powerful healing discipline. Because the lower potencies of 6 and 30 have no side effects when used responsibly and with respect, we can be confident that homoeopathic treatment for first aid and minor ailments is one of the safest and most effective forms of medicine. When homoeopathy is combined with a healthy lifestyle and naturopathic tips, we have a potent approach to holistic health care, both at the preventative stage and at the onset of minor problems. Good health is like inherited wealth. You do not fully appreciate its value and how difficult it is to reacquire it from scratch until you lose it!

## Regenerative Powers

There is also another subtler dimension to consider. Because homoeopathic remedies are so intimately connected with nature, like all forms of natural medicine, they have the ability to tap into nature's power. Their purpose is to re-establish harmony or homoeostasis in the body. This healing process is a mirror to nature's own self-regulatory and regenerative powers which are always attempting to reintroduce harmony and balance. When we pollute our seas with untreated waste, for example, nature's reaction is to attempt to step up the cleansing process by producing micro-organisms to ingest the pollutants. There is a force at work which acts to heal, regenerate and allow life to thrive. Many people now recognise this restorative, self-regulating organism at work as a planetary whole and call it 'Gaia'.

The curative processes at work in homoeopathy, and natural medicine generally, are like reflections of Gaia and are part of a larger whole. This medicine is in sympathy with our planet. It does not require that we plunder nature's resources to produce costly drugs or complex machinery. The remedies, taken from the animal, vegetable and mineral kingdom, are fundamentally benign and they create no harm. The manufacture of these remedies is also non-polluting, highly economical and long-lasting. They are also not tested on animals. Few synthetic drugs, many of which require complex chemical processes and all of which are tested on animals, can claim to have these advantages.

We began this final chapter in Section One by saying that natural medicine is a marriage of ancient and modern. This union of old knowledge and innovation is part of an evolving consciousness which increasingly attracts all kinds of people. Now is the time to discover and practise new alternatives to the ways we heal ourselves, grow food, educate our children and live together. Simply, the society in which we live is not working. Hospital and dole queues are growing whilst our social, educational and global resources are dwindling.

## Empowerment

The growing popularity of homoeopathy in Britain and the world at large is a testimony to this positive power of change. Human beings are capable of great insights and great personal qualities. If every aspect of our lives is handed over to the 'experts', we diminish our ability to find and develop those skills and attributes. It has never been our intention to denigrate the important role of doctors and professional practitioners. Instead, our aim is to open up a world of simple self-treatment which enables ordinary people to heal themselves naturally and in accordance with holistic principles. By learning this system of healing and by putting it into practice, you are becoming part of a larger process of self development and personal empowerment. You are also creating choices which may ultimately affect the way you view yourself and the world in which you live.

# SECTION TWO

## Prescribing

## The Art
## of
## Barefoot  Homoeopathy

# Chapter 7

# HOW TO PRESCRIBE
# THE BAREFOOT WAY

### The Shape and Form
### of Homoeopathic Remedies

The potencies suggested here can be given in the form of medicated pills or granules. The pills are made with a milk and sugar combination which is called *sac lac*. If they are very hard they can be chewed after a few minutes. The granules are made of pure sugar. One pill or a few granules should be placed on the tongue and allowed to dissolve in the mouth. In addition to pills and granules, homoeopathic remedies come in many other shapes or forms. There are powders (again *sac lac*) and liquid potencies for babies (although a pill can be crushed to a palatable powder between two clean spoons).

Homoeopathic remedies can also be made into creams, ointments and sprays. All three are used directly on the skin. *Pyretheum* spray is applied to stings. *Arnica* ointment is very good in the treatment of bruises and a mixture of *Calendula* and *Hypericum* in ointment form is excellent for cuts and sores.

### How to Care For Homoeopathic Remedies and
### Biochemic Tissue Salts

Homoeopathic remedies and biochemic tissue salts require special handling and storage so that they do not lose their power and become inert as a result of contamination. They should always be kept in the container in which they are supplied and never transferred to any other box or bottle which may have contained other substances.

They should be kept away from strong light, from great heat and especially from exposure to strong odours or perfumes, for example camphor, menthol, eucalyptus, moth balls or carbolic soap. Beware of keeping remedies continually in a car where the temperature can fluctuate greatly between extreme heat and cold.

If stocks of remedies are kept in corked or screw-top phials or bottles it is important never to uncork or uncover more than one remedy at a time. Neglect of this precaution could entail the risk of cross-potentisation and spoiling the remedies. Also the container should be uncorked or unstoppered for the minimum amount of time and care taken not to allow contamination of the cork or cap before replacement.

The medicine, i.e. a single dose, should be transferred directly from the cap to the mouth without touching hands or lips. Should you need to use your hands make sure that they are clean but free from all odours including soap. There is no need to wash the remedy down with water as absorption takes place in the mouth. Because remedies are absorbed in the mouth, it is a good idea not to take a remedy within half an hour of eating, drinking, smoking or brushing your teeth. Peppermints, lozenges, coffee and other strong flavoured substances should generally be avoided whilst on a course of homoeopathic remedies.

## How to Prescribe Homoeopathic Remedies for First Aid or Acute Conditions

Because this book is based on simple, common and non life threatening complaints, we only need to find two or three leading (i.e. most important) symptoms which match up to the remedy. These may be: 1) aching limbs; 2) a fever; 3) frequent sneezing. If, after turning to the appropriate section, the remedy is not immediately obvious, you can consider remedies listed under other ailments.

For example, a person has 'flu but may also have a splitting headache. He or she is unsure as to which remedy to choose having consulted the section relating to influenza. They should then turn to the section devoted to headaches and confirm the selection of the remedy by matching the symptoms to the appropriate remedy for their headache in that section. In the same way, another 'flu sufferer may have an upset tummy which troubles him or her more than aching limbs. This person should refer to the section on the stomach if the influenza section does not immediately yield the right remedy. Additionally, there may also be a common link between the two sections which will confirm that the original choice is indeed the correct remedy.

The book divides illnesses into categories to make prescribing simple for the reader. This is a convenience to help you find your way around. If, however, you have a migraine, for example, with both head pain with nausea and vomiting, you will need to decide which symptoms are uppermost and refer to the relevant section. Arrange the symptoms in order of importance, whatever the ailment may be, and start looking for the remedy which relates closely to the most important symptoms. Remember that homoeopathy is primarily concerned with the individual and not with the category of disease.

Once a remedy has been chosen, turn to the *materia medica* in Appendix 1 (page 153) if you wish to double-check your selection. This mini *materia medica* gives an overall 'picture' of the primary symptoms characteristic of each remedy. Cross-referencing in this way will help you to confirm the choice of remedy that you have made from the main prescribing section of this book (Section Two).

## Principles in Barefoot Prescribing

Remedies used homoeopathically are easy to administer and rapid in their effect but they must be used in accordance with homoeopathic principles and with attention to the right dosage.

Only one remedy should be given at a time, two pills per dose, and only a limited number of doses which are enough to bring about relief. The doses must be adequately spaced, the interval between successive doses being in direct relation to the urgency of the situation.

When selecting a remedy for self-treatment or for a friend with a minor ailment, there are certain rules of thumb. For an ailment like diarrhoea which has only recently affected the patient, 3 to 4 doses of the correct 30c remedy should show an improvement within hours. For a deeper complaint like indigestion or a sore throat, 24 to 36 hours should show an improvement. When prescribing for constipation, 2 to 3 days will be required before the efficacy of the remedy is displayed. Therefore, be patient when prescribing remedies for longer term acute problems like mild constipation. Give the remedy at night and in the morning for 3 days and not every hour as you would for sickness and diarrhoea. Again, **prescribe according to the urgency of the situation!**

Prescribing for chronic conditions, on the other hand, may require continued repetition of a remedy over a prolonged period. This should only be carried out by a professional homoeopath.

## The Golden Rule

The golden rule is always to stop the administration of the remedy when relief is obtained. **Repeat the remedy only if the symptoms return and do not use a remedy for more than 3 days.** This is important because there have been cases when sensitive people have felt unwell after prolonged use of homoeopathic remedies.

If the remedy has not helped you or the patient, then it is the wrong remedy and you should think again. Look for the changes. You would change the remedy if you are treating a nosebleed and it has not worked quickly. With a longer term ailment like constipation or boils for example, you would give its curative action more time to appear. You should never continue with a remedy, either after it has worked and you are better, or if it has not worked for you. Furthermore, the prolonged use of a remedy is unnecessarily wasteful.

## The Law of Cure

Remedies work according to observed processes or 'laws' developed by the homoeopath Constantine Herring. His law of cure can often be observed at work in acute prescribing and is described thus:

*From above to below*
*From within to without*
*From the centre to the circumference*
*From major organs to minor organs*
*Symptoms disappear in the reverse order of their*
*appearance.*

Patients who have taken to their beds often go to sleep after they have taken a remedy. Sleep is the most common amelioration witnessed and is a good indication that the right remedy has been chosen. Another homoeopathic phenomenon is witnessed when a rash begins in the upper part of the body and moves downwards until it is gone. *(From above to below.)* In the case of the after effects of tainted food, a patient may experience tummy pain and, on taking a remedy, open his or her bowels and feel better. *(From within to without.)* In measles, the cough comes first and is the last to go and the rash arrives last and goes first as the patient becomes well. This is a clear example of the law: *In reverse order of their appearance.*

In cases of chronic disease the patient will retrace the pattern that the disease has travelled and in doing so will experience the various ailments from which they have suffered in the past until they return to the condition from which the troubles began. **This is a long term phenomenon and does not apply to acute prescribing.**

You will note that this book is presented chapter by chapter, descending down the body, in a way that mirrors these principles of cure: the mind, the head, the chest, the stomach etc... This is to reflect homoeopathic principles and philosophy at work. Our aim is to introduce this fascinating world of medicine which encompasses the whole human being and not just his or her parts. The deeper holistic prescribing of practising homoeopaths takes into account the subtler aspects of people; their thoughts, feelings and aspirations first and then their physical concerns. Although simple home prescribing does not delve into these deeper questions, it is always beneficial to be mindful of the potential of homoeopathy. Who knows, your interest may take you further than the confines of this book!

# THE REMEDIES USED IN THIS BOOK
*(see Appendix 1 for a full description of each remedy)*

## Homeopathic Remedies (6c & 30c)

ACONITE *
AESCULUS
ALLIUM CEPA
ALUMINA
ANT TART
APIS *
ARG NIT
ARNICA *
ARNICA Ø
ARS ALB *
BELLADONNA *
BRYONIA *
CALC CARB *
CALENDULA
CALENDULA Ø
CANTHARIS
CAUSTICUM
CHAMOMILLA
CHINA
COCCULUS
COFFEA
COLOCYNTH
DROSERA
EUPHRASIA
EUPHRASIA Ø
GELSEMIUM *
GLONOINE
GRAPHITES *

HAMAMELIS
HAMAMELIS Ø
HEPAR SULPH *
HYPERICUM
HYPERICUM Ø
IGNATIA *
IPECAC
LACHESIS *
LEDUM
LYCOPODIUM *
MERCURIUS
NAT MUR
NIT AC
NUX VOM *
PETROLEUM
PHOSPHORUS *
PHYTOLACCA
PHYTOLACCA Ø
PULSATILLA *
RHUS TOX *
RUTA GRAV
SEPIA *
SILICA
SULPHUR *
SYMPHYTUM
THUJA
THUJA Ø
URTICA URENS

**Biochemic Tissue Salts (6x)**

CALC FLUOR *          KALI SULPH *
CALC PHOS *           MAG PHOS *
CALC SULPH *          NAT MUR *
FERR PHOS *           NAT PHOS *
KALI MUR *            NAT SULPH *
KALI PHOS*            SILICA *

 * Denotes remedies used most frequently in this book.
 Ø Denotes remedies applied in tincture form.

All the biochemic tissue salts are also available as homoeopathic remedies. They are made differently and, whereas homoeopathy works on the more subtle energies of the body, the tissue salts act on a more physical/cellular level.

It is not necessary to own all of these remedies to use this book. The remedies marked with an asterisk are the ones that we recommend to start with because they appear most frequently. Homoeopathic remedies last for years when stored correctly. Samuel Hahnemann's original remedies are still potent almost 250 years after they were made. There is nothing to stop a homoeopathic enthusiast acquiring a good home pharmacy in time!

**Naturopathic Tips**

Naturopathy is in essence a means of treatment which seeks to adjust the state of one's disorder by any substance which is natural to the body, i.e. foodstuffs, water, sun, air... Naturopathy regulates our health only through natural sources.

A few examples:
        Hot and cold water hip baths for haemorrhoids.
        Ginger for indigestion and nausea.
        Boiled oranges for constipation.

Throughout this book, we give naturopathic tips for many common ailments. This advice can be used in tandem with homoeopathic remedies, enriching your knowledge of natural medicine and making the process of treatment more effective.

## Common Sense

Like all ways of improving health, any recommended advice must be used with common sense and in moderation. Recently, comfrey came under the public eye because it was said to be toxic. It was fed in massive doses to mice who subsequently developed cancer. There was an argument as to whether it should be taken out of the health food shops and made into a restricted medicine. It seems obvious that if you feed paracetamol or aspirins to mice in large doses they will die, yet these are readily available, not only in chemists but in general stores throughout the country. Why then is comfrey such an evil?

In the same vein, a few years ago carrot juice received much publicity as a marvellous source of vitamins A and D. One individual drank so much that he turned orange and became very ill and died. Should carrot juice then be restricted on prescription?

With any form of medicine, common sense is a necessary attribute. All medicinal substances from homoeopathic remedies to vitamins and herbs must be treated with respect. It is unwise to binge on anything! The sensible maxim is 'moderation in all things'.

Homoeopathic philosophy is a fascinating subject and one that deserves detailed study but, as with most things in life, the test of a good dish is not so much in the recipe and method in which it is made but in the eating. The relief of discomfort and suffering with the use of homoeopathic remedies is where the value of this gentle and comprehensive system truly lies. The following chapters offer you the opportunity to test the recipe!

# Chapter 8

# MENTAL & EMOTIONAL PROBLEMS

There are situations with which we are all familiar that are not serious emotional or mental problems and can often be treated successfully with homoeopathic remedies. These include driving test nerves, stage fright, visiting the dentist, exam nerves, anxiety prior to operations, a sense of loss, sadness, nervous anticipation and over-excitement.

The most important consideration when prescribing homoeopathic remedies for emotional and mental complaints is how the person is **feeling**. When looking for the right remedy, categorise the symptoms in order of importance. For instance, the sufferer may be feeling sad but has an overwhelming sense of fear. You would therefore choose a suitable remedy which primarily treats fear rather than sadness.

Besides using remedies to help with mental and emotional complaints, there are many techniques which can specifically help these problems and strengthen our weaknesses. These techniques include relaxation exercises, the setting and achieving of 'goals', visualisation, daily positive affirmations and self hypnosis, or even walking the dog! The regular practice of yoga is also very helpful both as a complete form of exercise and an aid to relaxation. Many mental and emotional problems can be greatly helped by rest, relaxation techniques, a good diet and sensible exercise. Please refer to Chapter 5 which describes good 'lifestyle management' in detail.

Each person has a preference, or preferences, to different ways of combating anxiety, stress, depression and so on. What is important is to find out what is effective for you and practise it. Negative emotional states can be deeply paralysing. If emotional and mental distress continues or is a long term problem, please consult your practitioner.

# Anxiety, Anticipation, Shock & Lack of Confidence

ACONITE

Great anxiety.
Agonising fears with restlessness which accompany almost every ailment.
Fear of death, crowds, the future.
Agoraphobia.
Anxious, excited and nervous,
i.e. of impending operation, dental treatment.
Cannot sleep, tosses about.

ARG NIT

Nervous, impulsive and hurried.
Dreads ordeals.
Fear of crowds, high buildings, the dark.
Fear of business, of exams.
Over-anxious from too much study.
Fear of failure.

ARNICA

After a shock.
Wants to be left alone.
Mentally prostrate and apathetic.
Morose.
Says nothing ails them.
Hopeless and indifferent.
Feels good for nothing.
Agoraphobia.

ARS ALB

Oversensitive.
Anxious.
Despairs of getting well.
Fear of death.
Very restless.
Fear of being alone.
Fear of ghosts, burglars in the home, etc.
Demanding mentality.
Fussy.

CALC CARB

Doubting mood.
Fears diseases, misery, disasters and being observed.
Fear made worse from reports of cruelty.
Easily frightened and timid of everything.

GELSEMIUM

Afraid of falling.
Dread of ordeals.
Desire to be quiet and to be left alone.
Dullness, listless, languor.
Stage fright.
Bad effects of exciting news (especially in children), fright or fear.

LACHESIS

Very talkative.
Jealous.
Suspicious.
Restless, uneasy.
Mental energy best at night.
Very irritable if woken suddenly from sleep.

LYCOPODIUM

Confusion over daily affairs.
Afraid to be alone, of men, of own shadow.
Fear of new persons, having to perform in public.
Great loss of self-confidence.
Apprehensive.
Fear of breaking down in public.
Stage fright, but performs well once on stage.

NUX VOM

Active, angry or impatient people.
Very irritable when unwell or out of sorts.
Worse for noise, odours, overindulgence.
Sullen and fault finding.
Business stress and worry.
Worse for extreme overwork.
Shock.

PHOSPHORUS
Anxiety of being alone at twilight, ghosts, thunderstorms, the future.
Quickly prostrated by unpleasant impressions.
Very sensitive to impressions.
Pleading and whining.

PULSATILLA
Mild, timid, emotional people.
Very tearful.
Fear of the opposite sex.
Fear of being alone, the dark, ghosts.
Unorthodox religious ideas.
Craves sympathy and attention.
Suspicious and irritable

SILICA
Faint hearted, anxious, nervous, excited.
Lacks confidence.
Prostration of mind and body.

SULPHUR
Busy mind, lazy body.
Loves thinking, planning.
Full of ideas but relies on others to carry out the actions.

*Tissue Salts*

CALC PHOS
Anxious about the future.

KALI PHOS
Anxious, nervous.
Nervous when meeting people.
Nervous temperament.
Sensitive people.

## Sadness & Despondency

A naturopathic tip for overcoming the 'blues', anger or just generally feeling fed up is head bathing. Hold the head under a cold tap. The cool water turns a morbid state of mind into hopefulness!

ARG NIT

Loss of ambition.
Melancholic.
Despondent.
Irrational.
Believes they are despised by their family; that all their undertakings will fail.
Time passes slowly.
Wants to do things in a hurry.

ARNICA

Mentally prostrate and apathetic.
Morose.
Says nothing ails them.
Hopeless and indifferent.
Feels good for nothing.

ARS ALB

Melancholy.
Suspicious.
Fastidious.
Fault finding.
Increasingly irritable.
Groans, moans and weeps during their periods.

CALC CARB

Depressed.
Melancholic.
Doubting moods.
Sad and apathetic.
Desires to weep, to go home.
Suspicious.
Inability to apply themselves; hopeless.

GRAPHITES        Sad, irresolute, hesitates at trifles.
                 Feels miserable and unhappy.
                 Dreads work.

IGNATIA          Ailments caused by grief, after losing
                 persons or objects that were very dear
                 to them.
                 Ailments caused by jealousy and
                 disappointed love, i.e. teenage traumas.
                 Non-communicative, sighing, silent
                 brooding.
                 Finally sleeps but feels wretched on waking.

LYCOPODIUM       Confusion over daily affairs.
                 So sensitive that they weep when thanked
                 or spoken to.
                 Loss of self confidence.
                 Awakes sad.
                 Weeps all day.
                 Sad one minute, cheerful the next.
                 Cheerful at work but saves airing all
                 troubles for home.

NAT MUR          Irritable over trifles.
                 Awkward, hasty movements.
                 Chronic effects of grief.
                 Will never cry in public.

PHOSPHORUS       Weary of life.
                 Will not work, study or converse.
                 Apathy, indifference even to own children.
                 Wants sympathy.
                 Timid and irresolute.

PULSATILLA       Easily offended.
                 Whining.
                 Craves attention, sympathy.
                 Easily moved to tears.
                 Very irritable, very touchy.

SEPIA

Easily offended and miserable.
Nervous so that they want to hold onto something or could scream.
Aversion to family, sympathy and company, yet dreads to be alone.
Sad and irritable.
Spells of weeping.
Feelings altered by childbirth, menopause and premenstrual syndrome.

*Tissue Salts*

CALC PHOS

Peevish and fretful children.
Depressed spirits.
Desires solitude.
Poor memory and mind wanders from one subject to another.
Cannot concentrate thoughts.

KALI PHOS

Fatigued brain from overwork.
Depressed, gloomy, nervy people.
Homesickness.

MAG PHOS

Poor memory.

NAT MUR

Melancholy, hopelessness with dejected spirits.
Despondent moods.
Sleepy.
Weeps easily but usually when alone.

NAT SULPH

Feels discouraged.

## Effects of Bad News & Fright

ACONITE          Long term effects of fright.
                 Problems arising after surgical shocks or
                 injury.
                 From the acute attacks of fear.

GELSEMIUM        From depressing emotions, bad news,
                 unpleasant surprises.

IGNATIA          Ailments from grief, after losing persons or
                 objects that were very dear to them.
                 Also from jealousy and disappointed love.

# Acute Sleeplessness
# (short term insomnia)

Sleeplessness can be caused by worry, anxiety, overwork or an inability to 'switch off' at night. Relaxation exercises before going to bed are very helpful. It is also important not to drink tea and coffee in the evenings and not to overeat. A full stomach, particularly when it contains rich food, makes sleep very elusive. Fresh air is very soporific. A walk a day will aid sleep.

ARS ALB — Disturbed, anxious, restless.
Cannot settle the mind.
Wakes after midnight.
Disturbed dreams.

COFFEA — Nervous sleeplessness from rush of ideas, mental activity, drinking too much coffee, exhaustion.
Wakes at every sound.

NUX VOM — Gets to sleep but wakes early and cannot get to sleep again.
Finally sleeps but feels wretched on waking.

SULPHUR — Drowsy by day (cat naps), wakeful at night.
Talks, jerks and twitches during sleep.

*Tissue Salts*

KALI PHOS — Sleeplessness from nervous causes or over-excitement.

NAT PHOS — Sleeplessness due to digestive disturbances.

# Chapter 9

# THE HEAD

## Headaches

There are many reasons why people suffer from headaches, especially if they recur regularly. It is important to try and identify exactly why a person suffers from them and prevent or treat the underlying cause, rather than just taking remedies to treat headaches once they appear. These causes can include: mental tension, overwork, eye strain, lack of sleep, poor light and ventilation, overuse of VDU screens, dietary excesses (like too much chocolate!), hangovers, constipation, dehydration, misaligned spine, indigestion, bad teeth, and sinusitis.

On the dietary side, headaches and migraine attacks can be triggered by an intolerance to certain foods. These can include: pork, eggs, milk, cheese (and other dairy products), chocolate, cola, onions, garlic, citrus fruit, all alcohol (especially champagne and red wine), wheat, coffee, pickled herring, canned figs and broad bean pods! We can establish which food or foods are triggering headaches by refraining from eating them for a week and then introducing them into the diet. If they trigger the problem again, they are usually the culprit. It is interesting to note that a course of homoeopathic treatment with a practitioner can strengthen the constitution and, in some cases, make the patient more tolerant to the foods that trigger headaches.

Do you drink coffee or tea each morning to get you up and out to work and then discover that you get a headache at weekends if you sleep in for an extra hour or so? It seems that your body can become addicted to the caffeine contained in the drink which tends to constrict blood vessels. Apparently, without the daily jolt of caffeine, the blood vessels in the head dilate and this can cause head pain.

Headaches are often a message from the body, telling you that all is not well. Try to link up with the cause and eliminate it. When headaches do occur regularly and there is no simple reason such as an excess of caffeine, consult your practitioner for advice and treatment.

ACONITE

Sudden violent headaches, as if the skull contents would be forced out of the forehead.
Much throbbing in the temples.
Restless, anxious and thirsty.
Fullness, heavy, hot, bursting feeling.

APIS

Stinging, stabbing, burning pain.
Head feels bruised and tender all over.
Worse for heat, warm room, hot bath etc.
Better for cold in any form.
Brain feels tired.
Better for pressure.

ARG NIT

One sided headache.
Head feels too large.
Better for applying pressure.
Worse for motion and mental effort.
Caused by prolonged study or exertion, i.e. aerobic-type exercise.

ARNICA

Hot head with cold body.
Sharp pinching pain.
Scalp feels tight.

BELLADONNA

Violent, throbbing, hammering headache.
From catarrh.
Worse in forehead and temples.
Scalp very sensitive.
Worse for the slightest movement, bright lights, noise.
Generally worse on right side.
Better for firm pressure.

BRYONIA

Bursting, splitting, crushing pains.
On attempting to sit up feels sick and faint.
Worse for the slightest movement.
Better for resting and cold drinks.

GELSEMIUM

Occipital (back of head) headache.
Great heaviness of eyelids and limbs.
Blurred vision.
Hammering in base of brain.
Dull, heavy headache preceded by disturbance of vision.

GLONOINE

Waves of bursting, throbbing pain.
Face purple or scarlet.
Worse for heat, and every pulse beat.
Better lying down with head high.

NAT MUR

Throbbing, hammering, blinding headache.
Worse in the morning and in the evening.
Worse after a period.

NUX VOM

As if a nail were being driven into the skull.
Nausea and sour vomiting.
After effects of over indulgence in food or alcohol.
Hangover-type headache.
Frontal congestive headache linked to stomach.

PULSATILLA

Periodic headache from overwork or indigestion.
Pulsating, bursting pains, head feels very heavy, cannot raise head.
Better for fresh air.
Worse for rich foods, stuffy atmospheres.
Pressure on vertex (top of head).
Scalding tears from the eye nearest the pain.

SILICA

Headache from fasting or for not eating at the correct time.
Pain begins at back of head and settles over the eyes.

*Tissue Salts*

CALC PHOS

Headache with cold feelings in the head.
Worse for heat or cold.

CALC SULPH

Headache with vertigo and nausea.
Pain around whole of the head.

FERR PHOS

Headache from cold or sun.
Throbbing in temples or over eyes.
Congestive headache during the menstrual period.
Better for cold pack.
Worse for move

KALI MUR

Headache with vomiting.
Disordered stomach.
Sluggish liver.
Tongue coated white.

KALI PHOS

Headache from studying, nervousness, fatigue or anxiety.
Better for gentle movement.

NAT SULPH

Sick headache with biliousness.

# THE EYES

Eyes are very delicate organs. If a piece of grit or some such foreign body enters the eye, do not attempt to remove it by hand. Instead, flush it out with an eyewash. We recommend *Euphrasia* tincture in an eye bath. Make sure that your hands and any utensil you use are scrupulously clean as eyes are easily infected. Mix 1 part of the tincture with 20 parts of water. If the mixture stings unpleasantly, add more water.

Cold tea bags or slices of cucumber placed on the eyes revive tired, sore eyes. Also, it is important to have your eyes tested regularly. Eye tests can reveal many health problems at an early stage as well as provide prescriptions for glasses.

## Conjunctivitis
## Discharges
## Impaired Vision
## Photophobia (sensitivity to light)
## Styes

ALLIUM CEPA    Streaming eyes and nose.
Bland discharge from eyes.

APIS    Swollen eyes that burn and sting.
Styes, photophobia (sensitivity to light).

ARG NIT    Eyes continually watering.
Constant blinking.
Acrid discharge.

ARSEN ALB    Much burning in the eye, irritating discharge.
Eyes swell.
Intense photophobia (sensitivity to light).
Relieved from warm compresses.

EUPHRASIA Ø
Externally in tincture.
1 drop of tincture to 20 of water; applied as an eye wash.
Eyes water all the time and swim with tears.
Constant blinking.
Discharge is burning and acrid.
Sticky eye gum.
Conjunctivitis.
Photophobia (sensitivity to light).

GELSEMIUM
Vision dim, eyeballs sore, especially on moving them.
Eyelids droop, feel very heavy.
Double vision.

PHOSPHORUS
Vision obscured by mist, or veil; red mist or black spots before eyes.
Eyes tire easily on use.
Sees better by shading eyes by hand.

PULSATILLA
Profuse yellow discharge.
Styes.
Worse in warm room.

RUTA GRAV
Weakness of vision with blurring.
Eyes ache while in use.
Eyes feel hot and burning.

*Tissue Salts*

FERR PHOS
Burning inflammation, painful and red.
Better for cold applications.

KALI MUR
Whitish discharge with sensation of sand in eye.

NAT MUR
Neuralgic (aching) pains with flow of tears.

NAT PHOS
Discharge yellow creamy matter.
Eyelids glued together on waking.

SILICA

Inflammation.
Yellow, creamy discharges.
Styes and small boils on and around the
eyelids.

# THE EARS

Ear wax can cause a reduction in hearing ability and inflame the ear. It can be removed by either of two methods. The first is special ear 'candles' developed by the Hopi Indians which are gentle and painless and create a pleasant, relaxing sensation. The second method is by a warm water syringe. This is painless but should be done by a practitioner. Earache can have many causes such as catarrh, excessive wax, boils and as a complication of fevers. A good way of relieving the discomfort is to warm salt, place it in a cotton bag and apply it to the ear. Warm the salt in an oven but be careful not to make it too hot! If the symptoms persist, consult your practitioner.

## Earache & Discharges

ACONITE — Onset of chill.
Violent pain, ears hot and painful, worse lying on the affected side.

BELLADONNA — When throbbing is the main feature with red hot face.
Often associated with sore throat and swollen glands.
Worse for application of heat, worse on or in the right side.

CHAMOMILLA — For the child who reacts angrily.
Severe pains.
General pain.

HEPAR SULPH — When there is pus forming, before it is discharged and may have started as a sore throat.

PULSATILLA            Catarrh in the eustachian tubes
                      (the passages, one either side, leading
                      from the throat to the middle ear) caused
                      from being chilled after being hot.
                      Worse for application of heat.
                      Worse for being in the wind.
                      Weepy, clingy child.

*Tissue Salts*

FERR PHOS             Inflammatory earache with burning
                      throbbing pain after exposure to cold or
                      wet.

KALI MUR              Earache with swelling of the eustachian
                      tubes (the passages, one either side, leading
                      from the throat to the middle ear).
                      Catarrhal inflammation of the middle ear.
                      White or grey furred tongue and swelling
                      of the glands.
                      Cracking noise in the ear when swallowing.
                      Principal remedy for deafness from
                      swelling of the external ear.

MAG PHOS              Sharp pain in or around the ear.

# THE NOSE

## Bleeding

ARNICA          Bruising and bleeding after injury.


BELLADONNA      Red face, throbbing headache and bleeding.

CALC CARB       Nose bleeds in children.

IPECAC          Profuse red blood.

PHOSPHORUS      Frequent and profuse nose bleeds.
                Oversensitive to smells.

*Tissue Salts*

FERR PHOS       Inflammation of the tissues in the nose.
                During feverish illnesses.

# Sinusitis

A steam bath can do much to help relieve the painful symptoms of sinusitis. Put boiling water in to a bowl, hold the head (draped with a towel) directly over the bowl and breathe in the steam. Olbas Oil can also be very effective in the relief of sinusitis, but beware, it has a strong smelling vapour, and can antidote any homoeopathic remedy that is being taken.

ACONITE  Pain at root of nose.
Acute sense of smell.

PHOSPHORUS  Bad catarrh.
Bleeding from the nose when blown.
Sneezing worse for odours and smoke.

PULSATILLA  Blocked right nostril.
Pressing pain at the root of the nose.

SILICA  Sensitive nasal bones.

*Tissue Salts*

FERR PHOS  Fever, congestion and throbbing pain in the sinus area.

KALI MUR  Thick, white discharge with stuffy head.
Pain in sinuses.

# Catarrh

ARS ALB
: Copious, burning, clear, watery discharge with chilliness.

CALC CARB
: Nostrils sore and ulcerated.
Yellow discharge.
Good for catarrh in older people.

NUX VOM
: Stuffy colds, snuffles after exposure to dry, cold atmosphere.
Snuffles in a new-born baby.

PHOSPHORUS
: Chronic catarrh.
Facial bones painful.
Handkerchief 'bloody'.

PULSATILLA
: Discharge clear yellow or green.
Worse in evening or night, stuffy rooms, for lying down.
Clears with fresh air.

*Tissue Salts*

CALC PHOS
: Good general remedy for catarrh.
Catarrh in anaemic people.

KALI MUR
: Thick, white discharge with white coated tongue and stuffy feeling in the head.

NAT MUR
: Watery, transparent, frothy discharges.
Loss of smell and taste.

## Colds

Colds can be a cleansing process and they often occur in springtime and in the autumn. They are the body's way of ridding itself of dead cells. Colds should never be suppressed by decongestants or aspirins. If you have a cold, take plenty of rest, eat a very light diet, especially fresh fruit, and drink freshly squeezed lemon with hot water and honey or rosehip tea. Garlic pearles are also excellent in the treatment of any infection.

ACONITE — In the very early stages.
On the first night.

ALLIUM CEPA — With sneezing and watering of eyes and runny nose.

ARS ALB — With watery catarrh and sore nostrils.
Nose colds which descend to the chest.
Cold sores in the nose.

GELSEMIUM — When the onset is rapid, with chills running up and down the spine.
Aching in all limbs with typical 'flu-like symptoms.

HEPAR SULPH — In later stages when the catarrh is thick and yellow.

MERCURIUS — With much sweating, salivation and thick catarrh.
Worse for both extremes of temperature.
Foul taste in mouth.
Tongue flabby, shows imprint of teeth.

*Contd...*

| | |
|---|---|
| NUX VOM | From exposure to dry cold.<br>Much sneezing and stuffed up at night.<br>Streams in warm room, better out of doors.<br>Extremely chilly, cannot get warm.<br>Cold and hot in turns.<br>Fits of sneezing after meals. |
| PHOSPHORUS | Begins in chest or throat; tight feeling in chest.<br>Hacking cough. |
| PULSATILLA | Persistent cold.<br>Thick, yellow, bland discharge.<br>Better for being outdoors. |

*Tissue Salts*

| | |
|---|---|
| CALC PHOS | For convalescing after a cold. |
| FERR PHOS | Beginning of a cold when there is feverishness, stuffiness and sneezing. |
| KALI MUR | White phlegm and stuffiness with congestion. |
| NAT MUR | Cold is watery, loose, accompanied by feelings of discomfort.<br>Dry skin, loss of taste and smell. |

# Hayfever

Hayfever is an unpleasant complaint and one that conventional medicine treats with drugs like antihistamine which make the sufferer sleepy. It mostly occurs in the summer months when the pollen count is high but can be triggered by any irritating substance. Homoeopathic remedies can be of great help to those suffering from hayfever-like symptoms. If they are acute 'one-off' symptoms caused by exposure to an irritant, it is possible to treat oneself. If the complaint is seasonal or long term, it is better to seek the advice of your practitioner. If you suffer from long term hayfever, a visit to your homoeopath before the onset of the symptoms is preferable. Do not wait until it is in full flight!

A useful tip is to shower the head in cold water after exposure to pollen or other irritants.

ALLIUM CEPA     Nose and eyes stream, sneezing is severe and of increasing frequency.
Nostrils and upper lip become sore.
Worse indoors, in the morning and from contact with flowers.

ARS ALB     Sneezing violent and painful.
Violent tickle at one particular point inside nose, not relieved by sneezing.
Profuse watery discharge which burns the lip.

EUPHRASIA     Much sneezing.
Discharge from the nose is bland, but is burning from the eye.
Throat is often involved with hard dry cough.
Worse for open air, wind, lying down.

*Contd...*

GELSEMIUM       Violent sneezing, nose streams worse in the
                morning and discharge feels like acidic
                burning.
                Eyes feel hot and heavy.
                Swallowing difficult.

NUX VOM         Prolonged distressing spells of sneezing.
                Nose runny by day and dry at night.

*Tissue Salts*

FERR PHOS       Congestion, inflammation and headache.
                Difficulty with breathing.

NAT MUR         After exposure to the sun.
                Generally watery symptoms with feeling of
                itching and tingling in the nose.

SILICA          Itching and tingling of nose with violent
                sneezing.

# Chapter 10

# THE THROAT & CHEST

## Sore Throats

Sore throats can be relieved temporarily by salt water gargles which are very antiseptic. It is also helpful to drink freshly squeezed lemons with hot water and honey to taste or an infusion of rosehip tea. Do not drink these immediately before or after a remedy. Red sage tea is also soothing for throat complaints. Infuse 2 teaspoons in half a pint of boiling water and leave to stand for 10 minutes. Gargle with this cooled mixture 3 to 4 times a day. A few drops of propolis tincture (available from health shops) in warm water is another good remedy to use in a gargle. Hot and cold compresses applied externally on the throat will treat inflammation and help with the pain (particularly useful to use on children when you cannot get them to gargle).

ACONITE — Burning, smarting, dryness with tingling in throat which is very red.
Sudden onset after exposure to cold winds.
Hurts to swallow.

APIS — Burning, stinging pains in throat which is swollen and soggy-looking.
Better for cold, worse for heat.
Absence of thirst.

BELLADONNA — Typical scarlet fever throat; dry and burning.
Tonsils inflamed and bright red.
Averse to taking fluids.
Red hot face and skin.

GELSEMIUM        Difficulty in swallowing, cold shivers up
                 and down spine.
                 Worse for damp weather.
                 Absence of thirst.

HEPAR SULPH      Infection with splinter-like sensation in the
                 throat.
                 High temperature.
                 Possibility of an abscess forming.

IGNATIA          Tonsils inflamed, hard and swollen.
                 White spots on the tonsils.
                 Stitching pain extending to the ears.
                 Painful glands, possible fever with red face
                 and little thirst.

LACHESIS         Painful swollen throat, worse on left side,
                 worse for drinking hot liquids but
                 swallowing of food is easier.
                 Pain worse on waking.
                 Throat is sensitive to touch; cannot stand
                 being touched by scarf or collar.

MERCURIUS        Painful, ulcerated throat.
                 Bad breath, stinging throat pains and
                 marked sweating with raised temperature.
                 Thick yellow coating on tongue.
                 Much salivation.

*Tissue Salts*

CALC FLUOR       Relaxed throat with tickling in the larynx.

CALC PHOS        Sore, aching throat.
                 Hurts to swallow.
                 Large, swollen tonsils.

CALC SULPH       Can prevent severe development of a cold
                 if taken in the early stages.
                 Good for ulcerated sore throats.

FERR PHOS        Hot throat with pain and dryness.
                 Inflammation and burning pain, throat red
                 and dry with hoarseness, loss of voice.
                 Over use of voice, for public speakers,
                 singers, etc.

KALI MUR         Throat ulcerated with whitish or greyish
                 patches.
                 Characteristic white tongue.

## Coughs

An infusion of red sage tea is an excellent aid to coughs. If you do not have any red sage in the house, ordinary sage is a good stand-by. Hot and cold packs applied alternately to the chest will aid coughs. When applying packs wrap the patient up well to prevent chills.

ACONITE         Constant short, dry cough, with feeling of suffocation.
Hard, dry ringing cough which is brought on by, or worse for, cold.
Worse at night.

ANT TART       Persistent cough with rattling respiration.
Great accumulation of sticky phlegm.
Great difficulty in expectorating (coughing up phlegm).
Sudden sensation of suffocation - must sit up.
Pale, sickly face.

ARS ALB        Wheezing respiration, much frothy phlegm, cannot breathe fully or freely.
Worse after midnight.
Very restless and anxious.
Marked weakness and exhaustion.
Worse for lying down.

BELLADONNA   Dry, tickling cough in violent spasms.
Dryness in larynx.
Child begins to cry before coughing fit comes on.

BRYONIA

Hard, dry, spasmodic cough, shakes the whole body.
Associated with stitches and soreness in chest.
Bursting headache.
Onset from dry cold weather.
Worse for coming into warm room, slightest movement, after eating and drinking.

DROSERA

Crawling in larynx which provokes coughing.
Violent tickling in the larynx which wakes the sufferer from sleep.
Spasmodic cough until sufferer retches or vomits.
Cough from deep down in the chest provoking pain and sufferer holds chest until cough stops.
Cough worse at night.

HEPAR SULPH

Suffocating coughing spells.
Worse in cold dry weather when body gets cold or uncovered and when breathing in cold air.
Better in warm moist weather.
Chilly and sweaty and thirsty for hot drinks.

IPECAC

Spasmodic, suffocating cough with rattling respiration early in illness.
Cough incessant and violent with each inhalation.
Wheezing with sensation of tightness in the chest.

NUX VOM

Violent cough with bursting headache.
Hoarse, dry throat.
Sensation as if something was torn in the chest by cough.

PHOSPHORUS    Hoarse, sore, painful larynx.
Dry, hard, hacking cough.
Cough from dry tickling in throat.
Sensation of weight on chest and tightness
across it.
Worse for moving from warm room into
cold air, talking, laughing.

PULSATILLA    Cough loose in the morning and dry in the
evening.
Must sit up in bed to gain relief.
Phlegm thick.
Worse in warm room, for lying down and
in evening.

SEPIA    Dry, very tiring cough which seems to come
from the stomach.
Rotten egg taste in the mouth.
Worse in the morning with lots of salty
phlegm.
*Sepia* is a good remedy for finishing off
whooping cough when it lingers.

## Whooping Cough

Whooping cough is a serious complaint in children but homoeopathic remedies can be very helpful in its treatment. Homoeopathy can also provide preventative (prophylactic) treatment for parents who do not want, or indeed cannot have, their child vaccinated. We suggest that you seek the advice of your practitioner in the prevention and treatment of this complaint.

# Chapter 11

# THE ABDOMEN

## Stomach Pain
## (Including indigestion & heartburn)

The stomach is a very sensitive organ connected to a large number of nerves. It is also a barometer of feeling. We feel emotions 'in the pit of the stomach'. We have 'sinking feelings' and can't 'stomach' certain things, especially if we are 'yellow bellied'! Consequently, when we are unhappy or under stress, tummy symptoms can come to the fore. Therefore, if you experience stomach cramps, indigestion and heartburn regularly, a review of your lifestyle and aspirations may be helpful.

In the short term, slippery elm powder made with milk or preferably soya milk is a soothing and gentle drink. It neutralises acid in the stomach and aids digestion. It is also very nutritious. Herb teas containing chamomile, peppermint and marshmallow are far better than tea and coffee which is very harsh on the stomach and can aggravate the discomfort. Spicy and rich foods, too much alcohol, excessive sugar and smoking also aggravate the stomach. By contrast, a few cardamom or fennel seeds chewed after a meal aid digestion.

To improve digestion, meals should be small and frequent, possibly even 6 times daily and food should always be chewed extremely well.

An excellent remedy for indigestion and nausea is root ginger tea. Grate a small amount of fresh ginger and infuse in boiling water. Add honey to taste.

ARG NIT
Pain occurs in small spot and radiates
in all directions.
Ulceration of stomach.
Eating aggravates stomach pains,
particularly sugar and alcohol.
Constricted wind.
Stomach trembles and throbs.
Nervous indigestion.

ARS ALB
Burning pain in the stomach.
Better for warm milk.
Craves sips of ice cold water which may be
vomited immediately.
Loss of appetite with thirst.
Anxiety felt in pit of stomach.
Heartburn.

COCCULUS
Bloated abdomen and sensation as if full of
sharp stones when moving.
Complete loss of appetite.

COLOCYNTH
Stomach cramps.
Cutting pain in abdomen which is better for
bending double and for hard pressure.
Pains in waves.

LYCOPODIUM
Burning belches.
Eating small amounts creates fullness.
Cabbage, oysters and beans disagree.
Gnawing pains better for drinking hot water.
Desires sweets, pastries.
Preference for hot food.

NUX VOM
Heartburn.
Food lies like a heavy knot in stomach.
Stomach bloated and sensitive to pressure.
Craves rich food, alcohol and other
stimulants which aggravate.
Indigestion from drinking strong coffee.

PHOSPHORUS    Pain in stomach, better for cold drinks.
              Stomach ulcers.
              Burning pains, worse for eating.
              Craves cold drinks, salt, acid and spicy
              things.

PULSATILLA    With nausea and heartburn.
              Worse for fatty foods.

SULPHUR       Burning belches.
              Drinks a lot and eats little.
              Worse for eating.
              Worse at night.
              Suddenly hungry and weak at 11 a.m..

*Tissue Salts*

MAG PHOS      Sharp, cramping pains.

NAT PHOS      Acidity, sourness.
              Sour belches.
              Caused by excess of sugar or milk.

## Nausea
## (including travel sickness)

Sea Bands are helpful in treating nausea. They are not only effective for the traveller, but they can also alleviate nausea caused by pregnancy and drug enduced nausea. They are elasticated bands that exert pressure on acupuncture points in the wrist.

ANT TART    Nausea which comes in waves with weakness and cold sweat.

ARS ALB    Worse after midnight.
Worse for ice-cream, ice cold drinks or watery fruits.
Worse for sight or smell of food.
Nausea caused by jet lag.
Nausea during pregnancy.

COCCULUS    Especially good for travel sickness, especially seasickness.

IPECAC    Constant nausea.
Good for travel sickness generally.

NUX VOM    Worse in morning as if suffering from a hangover.

PETROLEUM    Sensitivity to petrol fumes.

PULSATILLA    Better in the open air.
Lack of thirst.
Good for nausea during pregnancy.

# Vomiting

ARS ALB    Vomiting with diarrhoea.
Gastroenteritis.
After eating ice cream, icy drinks and
watery fruit.

IPECAC    When nausea persists after vomiting.

NUX VOM    Vomiting two hours after meals.
Indigestion with vomiting.
Vomiting caused by too many stimulants
(i.e. coffee, alcohol, drugs).
Hangover.

## Colic in Infants

Colic in babies usually occurs in the early months at a regular time each day. Colic is a broad term used to describe general spasmodic pains in the abdomen. Although distressing (and exhausting!) for the parent as much as for the baby, the infant grows out of it within a few months in most cases. It is more likely to occur in babies which are fed artificially and in such cases it will generally be found that a temporary change of diet will be necessary. Consult your health visitor if you are at all concerned.

CHAMOMILLA    Irritable, restless and cross.
Nothing will console child.
Better for being picked up and carried.
Worse at night.

COLOCYNTH    Cutting pains in abdomen.
Colicky pains which come in waves,
better for bending doubling and
hard pressure.

*Tissue Salts*

MAG PHOS    Spasmodic, darting pains.

NAT PHOS    A good acid neutraliser.

## Loss of Appetite

Going off one's food can be for many reasons. The following remedies are useful particularly when considered in conjunction with other symptoms of minor ailments from an upset stomach to 'flu.

CHINA               Stomach feels full all the time.
                    Aversion to all food.

IGNATIA             Appetite for a variety of foods but desire
                    vanishes when offered them.

LYCOPODIUM          Hungry yet full after a few mouthfuls.

NUX VOM             Sour, bitter belches.
                    Hungry yet unable to eat.

PULSATILLA          Little appetite and no thirst.
                    Sudden aversion to food.

## Abnormal Thirst

Craving for or an aversion to liquids can be for many reasons. The following remedies are useful particularly when considered in conjunction with other symptoms of minor ailments from an upset stomach to 'flu.

ARS ALB        Wants to drink little and often.
               Worse for icy cold drinks.
               Stomach settles after warm drink.

BELLADONNA     When the mouth is dry, hot and red.
               Desire for large amounts of cold water or
               lemonade.

BRYONIA        Thirst for large quantities of cold drinks.
               Desire for bitter drinks.

PHOSPHORUS     Thirsty for cold drinks which are soon
               vomited.

SULPHUR        Thirsty but not hungry at all.

# Haemorrhoids

Apply witch-hazel to the area on a cotton wool pad. Remember to keep the witch-hazel in the fridge. Alternate hot and cold hip baths are also helpful. Take a 15 minute warm/hot hip bath and then 5 minutes of cold water. Always finish with a cold hip bath and remember to shower the legs and the abdomen with cold water as well.

AESCULUS        Sharp shooting pains up the back.
                Painful, protruding or blind and bleeding piles.
                Worse for standing and walking.

HAMAMELIS       Internally by mouth in pill form.
                With soreness like a bruise.

HAMAMELIS Ø     Externally in tincture.
                1 drop of tincture to 10 of water.

HYPERICUM       Very sensitive and easy to bleed.

NIT AC          Painful piles which bleed easily.
                Rectum feels torn.
                Itching piles.

NUX VOM         Blind, itching piles.
                Bleeding better for cold bathing.
                Piles from chronic constipation.

SULPHUR         Piles during pregnancy.
                Piles external or internal that are sore, raw or tender, burn, bleed or smart.
                Redness around the anus with itching.
                Loose, frequent bowel motions.

## Itchy Anus

CAUSTICUM        Itchy anus.
                 Better for bathing with cold water.

GRAPHITES        Smarting, itching, sore anus.

IGNATIA          Itching anus, often with stitching pains.
                 Sensation can extend deep into rectum.

NIT AC           Anus itches and oozes moisture.

PETROLEUM        Itching of anus after stools.
                 Anal fissures.
                 Worse for travelling.

SULPHUR          Itching with redness around the anus.

## Diarrhoea

Mild diarrhoea is the body's way of ridding itself of toxins and unwanted matter. It is necessary to allow this process and not to suppress it. As with stomach pain, slippery elm helps to line the intestines and is a gentle, soothing drink. As much fluid is lost with diarrhoea, it is important that your liquid intake is maintained.

ARS ALB
: Severe diarrhoea as a result of taking spoilt food; may be accompanied by vomiting.
Severely weakened after each bowel movement.

BRYONIA
: Profuse diarrhoea which starts in the early morning.
May be as a result of drinking too much cold water.
Also as a result of hot weather.

CHAMOMILLA
: Diarrhoea in teething infants.
Stools may be grass green and contain particles of undigested food.
Diarrhoea smells like rotten eggs.

CHINA
: Debilitating, painless diarrhoea with offensive smell.
May result from summer chill or from eating too much fruit.

COLOCYNTH
: Frequent diarrhoea with colicky pains, better for pressure, i.e. bending double.
Stools are copious and thin, spluttery and yellow.

*Contd...*

GELSEMIUM        Diarrhoea from emotional excitement,
                 fright or bad news.
                 Stools painless and involuntary.
                 Cream or greenish in colour.

NUX VOM          Diarrhoea from over-indulgence.
                 May alternate with constipation.
                 Stools may contain mucous and blood.

PHOSPHORUS       Painless, exhausting diarrhoea.
                 Involuntary after fright.

PULSATILLA       Watery diarrhoea, worse at night.
                 From too much fruit.
                 From nervousness or fright.
                 Worse for rich, fatty food.

SULPHUR          Diarrhoea in early morning which is
                 painless and variable in consistency and
                 amount.
                 Offensive smell.

## Constipation

Constipation is caused by too little roughage in the diet, too little exercise, failure to acquire the habit or take the time to pass regular stools, too little fluids, pregnancy, or lack of tone of the colon muscle. Many people take extra wheat bran as a safeguard against constipation. This is alright in small doses, though an excess of bran creates phytic acid in the bowel which may actually contribute to digestive disorders. The best method is to eat unrefined foods regularly like wholemeal bread and brown rice and make sure you eat plenty of fresh vegetables and fruit. This is better than lots of bran at breakfast. Soaked prunes are also popular and effective as are boiled oranges.

Exercise is important and yoga is especially good as it stimulates the system and helps establish regular bowel motions. Finally, a regular time each day, set aside for bowel motion will re-establish the habit. Laxatives do nothing in the long term and are an artificial solution to an important health problem.

ALUMINA         Chronic inactivity of bowel.
                Great straining.
                Even a soft stool is very hard to pass.
                Dryness in rectum.

BRYONIA         Stools difficult to pass; large, hard and dry.

CALC CARB       Constriction in the rectum.
                Stools large and hard containing
                undigested food.
                May feel generally better when constipated.

GRAPHITES       Large, difficult, knotty stools.

LYCOPODIUM      Stools hard, small, difficult to pass and
                incomplete.
                Useless urging.
                Traveller's constipation.
                During pregnancy.

NAT MUR

Stools light, dry and crumbling.
Constipation every other day from
inactivity.

NUX VOM

Useless urging.
Small amounts passed at each attempt.
Feeling as if there is still fecal matter left in
the rectum.
Constipation caused by a bad diet.

*Tissue Salts*

NAT MUR

Small, dry, lumpy stools, caused by a
lack of moisture in the intestines.

# Chapter 12

# THE URINARY SYSTEM

## Cystitis, Irritable Bladder & Infections

When suffering from any form of urinary disorder, it is important to drink plenty of water and to avoid tea and coffee. Additionally, herb teas like chamomile and dandelion coffee are diuretics and create the urge to pass water and should be avoided, along with all citrus fruits. The liquid from boiled pot or pearl barley should also be drunk by the pint, but not the commercial barley water which contains sugar. Indeed all sugar should be avoided as it aggravates the bladder. 100ml of cranberry or cherry juice drunk 4 to 5 times daily will aid bladder conditions.

APIS
Burning and stinging pains while urinating; urine is scanty and concentrated.
Last drops burn.
Cystitis.
Difficulty passing urine when prostate gland is enlarged.

ARS ALB
Burning pain causes agitation; unable to keep still with pain.
Feeling of weakness in the abdomen after urinating.

BELLADONNA
Acute urinary infections.
Frequent and profuse urination.
Dark urine.

CANTHARIS    Frequency of urination with scalding pain.
             Cystitis.
             Kidney region sensitive.
             Intolerable urging but little is passed in drops.

GELSEMIUM    Profuse, clear watery urine with extreme
             chilliness.
             Retention of urine.

PULSATILLA   Increasing desire to urinate.
             Worse when lying down.
             Pain in bladder after urinating.

*Tissue Salts*

FERR PHOS    Constant desire to urinate.
             Hot and painful urination.

KALI MUR     Thick, white mucous in the urine.

## Incontinence

Incontinence in women, especially as a result of pregnancy, can be helped and even avoided by pelvic floor exercises. The sphincter muscles around the bladder can be toned up by simple exercises which can be practised anywhere, whether you are standing, sitting or lying down. Pelvic floor exercises are not only for pregnant women. It is never too late to start practising!

Imagine that you have a tampon in the vagina which is falling out. Tighten the muscles in that area. The muscles of the anus will also tighten up but concentrate your attention on the vagina more than the anus. Do not contract the tummy muscles or your bottom or hold your breath. Just tighten the muscles in the vagina and hold them for a few seconds. Then relax and let go. Do this ten times a session, three times a day and build up the time in which you hold the muscles contracted. Practised regularly, this simple exercise can prevent and help incontinence in women.

The remedies given below are as appropriate for men as for women. Urinary disorders in older men, however, are often due to problems with the prostate gland. Homoeopathy can help this condition, but we recommend that professional advice is sought.

If you suffer from incontinence, avoid drinking tea and coffee and replace them with water or diluted fruit juice. 100ml of cranberry or cherry juice drunk 4 to 5 times daily will aid bladder conditions.

APIS              As a result of coughing.

BELLADONNA        On lying down, when standing,
                  when sleepy during the day or at night.

CAUSTICUM         On coughing and sneezing, blowing the nose
                  and walking.
                  In old people who hardly feel the urine
                  passing.

PULSATILLA        During pregnancy, often whilst walking.
                  Generally on lying down, coughing,
                  sneezing or on breaking wind.

SEPIA             During sleep.

*Tissue Salts*

CALC PHOS         Bedwetting in young children and older
                  people; frequent urging to urinate.

FERR PHOS         Incontinence from muscular weakness.
                  Worse for coughing
                  Worse for standing.

KALI PHOS         From nervousness.

# Chapter 13

# WOMEN'S COMPLAINTS

Many women have benefited greatly from regular smear tests and check ups. Cervical cancer can be stopped in its tracks at a pre-cancerous and even early carcinogenic stage by laser treatment. Once it is established, the treatment involves surgery and is usually more debilitating and is less successful. It is very important to use the services on offer and keep an eye on your health. Similarly, regularly checking one's breasts for lumps is a good course of action.

## Mastitis

Mastitis is the inflammation of breast tissue and usually occurs whilst breast-feeding but it can be caused by lowered vitality or a blow to the breast. A good preventative measure is to massage a mixture of almond oil and lemon juice onto the nipple throughout the pregnancy.

Mastitis symptoms can be relieved by applying hot and cold packs (i.e. flannels) to the area. Place a hot pack on the breast for 10 minutes and then alternate it with a cold pack for 5 minutes.

ACONITE          In the early and acute stages.

BELLADONNA       When the breast is heavy, hard, red with
                 streaks radiating from the nipple.
                 Pulsating pains; worse for touch,
                 movement or jarring.

BRYONIA　　　　　When the whole breast is hot, painful and
　　　　　　　　　very hard.

PHYTOLACCA　　　Internally in pill form.
　　　　　　　　　For very sensitive and stony, hard breasts.

PHYTOLACCA ∅ Externally in tincture.
　　　　　　　　　1 drop of tincture to 10 parts water;
　　　　　　　　　applied to the inflamed area.

*Tissue Salts*

SILICA　　　　　　A good general remedy for mastitis,
　　　　　　　　　especially when breast is discharging.
　　　　　　　　　Helps break down lumps.

## Sore Nipples

CALENDULA ∅    Externally in tincture.
1 drop of tincture to 10 parts water;
applied locally where the skin is broken.

PHYTOLACCA ∅ Externally in tincture.
1 drop of tincture to 10 parts water;
applied to the inflamed area.

SULPHUR    Sore and chapped around the base with
burning and bleeding.

## Pre-Menstrual Syndrome

CALC CARB    Bloated feeling, tender breasts.
             Headaches, colic, chilliness, milky vaginal
             discharge.
             Melancholic.

GRAPHITES    Distinct increase in weight.
             Delayed menstruation with constipation.
             Vaginal discharge instead of menstruation.
             Sad, fearful and irresolute.

LACHESIS     When there is fluid retention and heaviness
             of breasts.
             Suspicious, jealous, nervous, or
             loquacious.

LYCOPODIUM   Cross and melancholic.
             Intellectual types.
             Withdrawn.
             Does not strike out.
             Menses can be suppressed for months.

NUX VOM      Very irritable, impatient and quarrelsome.
             Will strike out.
             Worse after the period.

PULSATILLA   Mild, timid and emotional people.
             Changeable.
             Very tearful and irritable.
             Painful breasts.

SEPIA        Depressed and irritable.
             Indifferent to family.
             Very sad.
             Weeps alone.

## Absence or Suppression of Periods

ACONITE            Suppression following exposure to cold or as a result of shock or fright.

BRYONIA            Suppression associated with headaches or vicarious discharges, i.e. nosebleed or vaginal discharge instead of period.

PULSATILLA         Suppression following getting wet feet. From nervous disability or anaemia. Suppression in adolescents.

SEPIA              Absent after stopping the Pill.

*Tissue Salts*

KALI SULPH         Scanty or suppressed period with fullness of abdomen.

NAT MUR            In young girls when periods do not appear.

CALC PHOS          Anaemia with suppression of periods.

# Period Problems

ARS ALB
Periods too early and too heavy.
Burning around the ovaries.
Pain like red hot wires.
Great feelings of fatigue.
Worse for slightest exertion and better in a warm room.

BELLADONNA
Cramping pains with early period and heavy flow of bright red blood.
Pains similar to pangs of childbirth and with pressure in the pelvis as if the contents would be expelled.

CALC CARB
Periods early, profuse and too long.
Over excitement brings on periods.

GELSEMIUM
Periods late and scanty.
Pains extend to back of hips.

LACHESIS
Pain in left ovary.
Periods too short and light.
Menstrual pain is relieved by the onset of period.

PULSATILLA
Very tearful.
Painful breasts.
Periods too late, scanty, thick and dark.

SEPIA
Periods too early with profuse flow.
Late and scanty after weaning or at puberty.
Dragging or bearing down feeling as if pelvic contents would fall out of the vagina.
Sharp, violent stitching pains.

*Tissue Salts*

FERR PHOS        Profuse and painful periods.

MAG PHOS        Periods are early, pains neuralgic and
                 relieved by pressure or locally applied heat.

NAT MUR         Fluid retention, irritability and sadness.

## Vaginal Thrush

The majority of women suffer from this complaint at one time or another in their lives. It is caused by a fungus which disturbs the flora in the vaginal and sometimes the anal area, both inside and/or outside. Symptoms range from a discharge which resembles curdled milk to itching, redness, soreness, and inflammation of the affected area. This complaint requires professional treatment and so we do not list remedies in this book. If, however, you suffer from thrush, you can take *lactobacillus acidophilus* tablets which are available from health shops. They replace natural flora in the gut and help to harmonise the system.

There are also preventative measures that you can take. It is well known that tight clothing, especially jeans, being overweight, perfumed soaps, bubble baths and oils, vaginal sprays and deodorants, nylon underwear, antibiotics and cleaning oneself after a bowel motion from back to front can cause thrush. Some women are also sensitive to certain spermicidal creams and jellies, the Pill and drinks such as red wine. Excessive sugar in the diet can also aggravate the condition.

Finally, if thrush recurs persistently, your partner should be treated, even if he uses sheaths. Men often carry the fungus but have no symptoms and so sexual contact re-infects the female partner. All cotton underwear, towels and clothing which touch the infected area should be washed in very hot water during treatment as the fungus can live on in material and then reinstate itself when the clothes or towel are used again.

## The Menopause

During the menopause it is very important to ensure that you have a healthy diet and do not drink too much tea or coffee. Regular exercise, however gentle in nature, will also be a great help.

BELLADONNA    Dryness and heat in vagina.
Menses increased, too early, too profuse.
Hot, red skin.
Flushed face.
Internal coldness and external heat simultaneously.

GLONOINE    Throbbing in head with flushing.
Congestion in head.
General flushing.

LACHESIS    Palpitations, hot flushes, haemorrhages, headaches, faintness.
Worse for tight clothing.

SEPIA    Very heavy irregular periods.
Sudden hot sweats with sinking or dragging down sensation in uterus or abdomen.
Angry, sensitive, easily offended and miserable.
Indifferent to loved ones.

SULPHUR    Hot, red flushes with offensive perspiration.
Vagina itches and burns.

*Tissue Salts*

CALC PHOS    General weakness.
Run-down condition.
Anaemia.

KALI PHOS    Nervousness, anxiety and irritability.

# Chapter 14

# BACKACHE
# GENERAL ACHES & PAINS

## Backache

Homoeopathy is a good complement to the manipulative therapies like chiropractic, osteopathy, the Alexander Technique and remedial massage. As many as 80% of us suffer from back pain at one time in our lives and 26 million working days are lost each year. Many of these sick days could be avoided with the help of natural medicine and gentle but strengthening forms of exercise such as yoga.

If you suffer from constant back pain, it is very important to establish the cause. It could be misalignment of the spine or a trapped nerve. A visit to a reputable, qualified practitioner in the manipulative therapies should reveal the cause and offer treatment. Homoeopathy can help to reduce inflammation and swelling and treat the problem from within. It is useful before and after manipulation. Additionally, pulled muscles can be simply treated with homoeopathy and rest. After recovery, a gentle course of exercise like yoga is advisable to strengthen the back.

ARNICA            If caused by injury, overlifting and strain.

BRYONIA           Pain in the small of the back, worse for
                  walking or turning.
                  Stitches and stiffness in small of back.
                  Painful stiffness in neck.
                  Worse for change in weather.

HYPERICUM         For spinal concussion, injury to coccyx
                  with radiating pain up spine and down the
                  limbs.

NUX VOM

Backache in lumbar region.
Pain worse at night in bed.
Has to sit up in order to turn over.
Burning sensation in spine.
Constipation and irritability are common.

RHUS TOX

Stiffness and pain in the small of the back.
Lumbago.
Stiff neck.
Better for motion, pressure, lying on a hard surface, bending backwards.
Worse for sitting and standing still.

RUTA GRAV

Low lumbar pain.
Better for lying on the back and for pressure.

SEPIA

Ache in lumbar region on walking.
Weakness in small of back.
Worse for stooping and kneeling.
Better for pressing back into something hard.

*Tissue Salts*

MAG PHOS

Cramping pains along the spine.

NAT MUR

Weak back, especially in people who have a lot of salt.
Pain better for firm pressure.
Worse in the morning.

## Sciatica

Sciatic pain is often felt in the buttocks, the back of the thighs and the outside and front of the leg. It can sometimes extend to the top of the foot. It is caused by a disturbance to the sciatic nerve in the lower part of the spine, usually, but not always, caused by a misaligned spine.

ARS ALB            Sciatica with burning pains.
                   Uneasiness or heaviness felt in the legs.

CHAMOMILLA         Pains are worse at night and with excessive
                   sensitivity to pain.

COLOCYNTH          Cramping pains in the hips.
                   Sciatic pain in left side.
                   Better for pressure and heat and worse for
                   gentle touch.

HYPERICUM          Pain which radiates up the spine and down
                   the thighs.
                   Sciatica due to injury.

RHUS TOX           Pains down the back of the thighs.
                   Worse for cold, damp weather and at night.
                   Better for motion.

RUTA GRAV          Pains from back down to the hips.
                   Worse for lying down, at night.
                   Better during the daytime.

*Tissue Salts*

MAG PHOS           Sciatica with spasmodic pains.

NAT SULPH          Pain unrelieved in any position.
                   Worse for getting up from sitting,
                   or turning in bed.

## Cramps

Cramps usually occur in the calves and the feet. The cause is unknown though there is a relationship with the circulation. A strong sea-salt foot bath relieves cramp in the lower extremities.

ARS ALB            Cramps in calves which have a burning
                   quality to them.
                   Restlessness.
                   Worse in the early hours, just after midnight.

GELSEMIUM          Cramp in muscles of forearm.
                   Writer's cramp.
                   Loss of power, of muscular control.

NUX VOM            Cramps in calves and soles.
                   Must stretch out feet to relieve.

*Tissue Salts*

CALC PHOS          Cramps with a feeling of numbness,
                   cold and as if parts are asleep.

MAG PHOS           General cramps.
                   Spasmodic contractions.
                   Radiating pains.

# Chapter 15

# THE SKIN

The skin is the outer organ of the body. As such, it is a good reflection of the health of the person. If the diet is bad, the skin usually suffers. The skin can also reflect embarrassment, anxiety and nervous tension. The most obvious effect is blushing, although many rashes and skin complaints can also be triggered by the emotions as much as by one's general health.

It is always better not to suppress skin problems as this sends the complaint within. Help nature to bring them out naturally. Homoeopathic remedies can do just this and self-treatment for simple skin conditions is the best solution. Steroid creams suppress skin problems and should be avoided. If your skin problem is more than a minor complaint, seek advice and treatment from a homoeopath.

For general skin health, there is a method called 'the salt glow'. Place a few handfuls of sea salt in a bowl and add water to moisten it. Then rub it all over the body and rinse off afterwards. This is not for those with a tender skin or for those suffering from skin disorders. Otherwise its tonic action is quite marked if kept up regularly.

# Itching

ARS ALB              Restlessness, chilliness and itching with a
                     burning quality.
                     Urticaria (also called nettlerash).


PULSATILLA           Urticaria (nettlerash) after rich food or
                     after diarrhoea.
                     Worse at night from the heat of the bed and
                     undressing.
                     Symptoms are variable and periodic.


SULPHUR              Burning itching and redness.
                     Worse for washing, scratching and woollens.


URTICA URENS  Intense itching or burning of skin, like that
                     of a nettlerash.
                     Prickly heat and hives.
                     Skin has raised, red blotches.


*Tissue Salts*

FERR PHOS            For hives or urticaria (nettlerash) when it is
                     accompanied by fever.


NAT MUR             Urticaria (nettlerash), caused by overheating.

## Cracked Skin

GRAPHITES    Dirty looking and horny-like skin which exudes a gluey moisture and bleeds easily.

NAT MUR    Greasy, oily, unhealthy skin.
Hangnails.
Dry eruptions, especially around fingernails and on the edge of hair and bends of joints.

PETROLEUM    Thick, dirty-looking eruptions often with harsh, hard, dry skin which tends to crack.

SULPHUR    Dry, scaly, unhealthy looking skin which is red and itchy.

*Tissue Salts*

CALC FLUOR    Chaps and cracks of the skin, particularly in the palms.

SILICA    Deep cracking at finger tips which fail to heal.

# Boils

Boils begin as a sore spot and become hard, painful and full of pus. It is important to keep them very clean as they are prone to infection. Boils can reflect a lowered state of health and a bad diet. If you suffer from boils, review what food you are eating and your intake of sugar and alcohol. Opt for more fresh fruit, fresh vegetables and fresh air!

BELLADONNA    Boils in which there is a great deal of redness and inflammation.
In early stages before pus has formed.

CALENDULA ∅    Externally in tincture.
1 drop of tincture to 10 of hot water; applied locally.

HEPAR SULPH    To mature the boil and bring it to a head.

HYPERICUM ∅    Externally in tincture.
1 drop of tincture to 10 of hot water; applied locally.
When the area is sensitive to touch and is in a place which affects the peripheral nerves, causing great pain.

SILICA    Boils and pustules that appear anywhere on the body.

*Tissue Salts*

FERR PHOS    In the first stage when there is heat, pain and possibly a fever.

SILICA    Brings boils to a head and helps them disperse.

# Warts

CALC CARB          Warts on the face and hands.

CAUSTICUM          Warts on the nose, fingertips and eyebrows.
                   Tendency to bleed.

NIT AC             Warts, large and jagged in appearance
                   which bleed on touch or when washing.

THUJA              Internally in pill form.
                   Good for all warts.

THUJA ⊘            Externally in tincture.
                   Applied undiluted directly to warts on all
                   parts of the body.

*Tissue Salts*

NAT MUR            Warts on the palms of the hands.

## Dandruff & Falling Hair

ARS ALB           Itchy scalp with dry scales.
                  Very sensitive scalp; cannot bear to brush
                  or comb hair.

GRAPHITES         Moist, crusty dandruff.

LYCOPODIUM        Flaking, scaling and a lot of dry skin.
                  Falling or prematurely greying hair.

PHOSPHORUS        Itching of scalp.
                  Hair can fall out from specific areas in large
                  bunches.
                  Dandruff is copious.

*Tissue Salts*

KALI SULPH        Moist, sticky and yellow crusts.
                  Copious scaling of the scalp.

NAT MUR           White scales on scalp with falling of the hair.

# Chapter 16

# COMMON INFECTIOUS DISEASES

## Chicken Pox

Chicken pox is one of the most contagious viruses of all and for the first 7 days after contact it is at its height of infection. It remains contagious until 7 days after the appearance of the rash or until all the vesicles (i.e. spots) are dry. The vesicles appear between 12 and 21 days after contact. Red spots appear on the scalp, face and body and then spread to the limbs. The temperature rises once the rash appears and then falls after a day or two. The spots then become blisters.

In children, chicken pox is a minor ailment. In adults, it is more unpleasant and often is accompanied by a high fever. The vesicles look like blisters and are very itchy. If they are scratched, they leave scars, especially on the face. To contain the itchiness, do not let the sufferer get too hot in bed and dress him or her in loose cotton clothing. Bathe the skin in tepid water and then apply calamine lotion.

ACONITE — Feverishness with symptoms of anxiety, fear, thirst, dry, heat, rapid, hard, throbbing pulse.

ANT TART — Helps development of vesicles when eruption is slow to form.

BELLADONNA — High fever, burning face, headache. Hot head, cold limbs.

LEDUM — Red spots and rash. Worse on covered parts.

RHUS TOX        The first remedy to be prescribed in the
                early stages.
                Restless in mind and body.

SULPHUR         Itchy skin.
                Worse in bed, scratching, washing.
                Hungry but eats little.
                Extreme thirst.

*Tissue Salts*

FERR PHOS       For feverishness, in early stages, before the
                vesicles develop.

NAT MUR         Chilliness, night sweats, headache with
                clear, watery vesicles.

## German Measles

German measles, termed medically as Rubella, is not a serious complaint, except in pregnant women. For this reason, it is given twice to children in a combined inoculation with measles and mumps (known as MMR), once in their first and again in their fifth year. German measles still occurs, however, either because a child has not been inoculated or because it is possible to contract it after inoculation.

It is caused by a virus and is infectious for 7 days before the rash appears and at least 4 days afterwards. The symptoms appear 14 - 21 days after contact. The rash begins on the face, scalp and body and spreads to the limbs and looks like small bumpy red spots. The symptoms begin with a sensation of mild discomfort and develops into a rash which resembles nettle-rash (urticaria). There is sometimes a runny nose and sore throat. There can also be swollen glands in the neck and behind the ears.

German measles does not endanger the sufferer but it is essential that pregnant women, in the early stage of pregnancy, avoid the disease at all costs as the virus can damage the unborn child.

ACONITE          Fever with anxiety, thirst and restlessness.
                 Rash is red, hot and burning.

BELLADONNA       Rash red, hot and dry.
                 Unaffected skin is pale.
                 Tender, swollen glands in neck.

BRYONIA          Rash slow to form and can disappear
                 suddenly.
                 Skin hot and swollen.
                 Pulse hard and quick.
                 Hot internally but feels cold externally.

*Contd...*

PULSATILLA        Chilliness, yet dislikes a warm room.
                  No thirst, even with a fever.
                  Changeable symptoms.
                  One part of body can be hot and another
                  chilly.
                  Erratic temperature.

URTICA URENS  Violent itching with burning heat.

*Tissue Salts*

FERR PHOS         Excellent generally, where there is a high
                  temperature, quick pulse and an inflamed
                  rash.

## Glandular Fever

Glandular fever is a complaint that conventional medicine cannot treat, nor can it predict how long it takes to recover from it. Glandular fever can have many symptoms including: sore throat; red cheeks; swollen glands in the neck, armpits and groin; raised fever; great exhaustion; depression; headaches; swollen joints, liver and spleen. In some cases the fever relapses again and again. It seems that adolescents are most vulnerable to it although it can affect people at any age.

When treating the acute stage of glandular fever, it is necessary to find out the most acute symptoms in each individual and treat them. For instance, is the person experiencing a terrible sore throat primarily or are the headaches uppermost? Is the fever most marked or are the swollen glands more relevant? Take the individual's uppermost symptoms.

Like any complaint, glandular fever can be severe or mild. If in doubt, consult your practitioner for treatment. Homoeopathy is also very effective in treating relapses and the long lasting effects of glandular fever, including mental symptoms like depression.

BELLADONNA Delirious with high fever.
Internal coldness with external hot, red heat.
Hot head with cold limbs.
No thirst.
Throat red, hot, swollen.
Worse on right side.

BRYONIA Heavy, crushing, bursting, or splitting headache.
Worse for moving eyes, coughing.
Fever with hot head and red face.
Worse in warm room.
Sour sweat.

GELSEMIUM      Tired, heavy limbed, weak with soreness.
               Aching all over.
               Chill up and down back.
               Can tremble.
               No thirst.

LACHESIS       Swallowing hurts.
               Worse for liquids, better for solids.

MERCURIUS      Easily chilled or overheated.
               Profuse sweat which brings no relief.
               Sour, unpleasant, sweetish or strong odour.

NAT MUR        Hammering, bursting, heavy headache
               over the eyes.
               Thirsty.

RHUS TOX       Sore throat with swollen glands.
               Tonsils can be yellowy.
               Easily chilled and worse if uncovered,
               accompanied by pain in limbs.

*Tissue Salts*

FERR PHOS      Excellent generally, where there is a
               high temperature and a quick pulse.

## Influenza

'Flu is very infectious and the incubation period can be between one to three days. 'Flu starts with a sore throat, a runny nose and a raised temperature. The limbs usually feel heavy and ache and the sufferer is alternately hot and cold and shivers. There is a loss of appetite, possibly vomiting and a headache. The illness can go on from two days up to a week. It may leave the sufferer with a great feeling of weakness and even sinusitis.

It is wise to go to bed and rest with 'flu. Antibiotics do not affect the virus but homoeopathic remedies can ease the symptoms. Eat a light diet, keep warm and drink plenty of fluids.

Because there are a number of 'flu viruses, it is not always possible to take the correct homoeopathic 'flu prevention. Many people do, however, find special homoeopathic preparations helpful in the prevention of 'flu. Additionally, health shops do sell commercially prepared homoeopathic remedies to ward off 'flu and people do find they work.

A word of warning: influenza can be a very serious complaint, especially in the very young, the frail and the elderly. Please seek medical help immediately if they are in one of these vulnerable categories.

ACONITE         In early stages with fever with cold sweats and alternating hot and cold sensations.

ARS ALB         Exhaustion, weakness and prostration, chilliness and restlessness with anxiety.
Burning pains are characteristic.
Burning nasal discharge with sneezing and conjunctivitis.
Thirsty.
This remedy is well indicated when diarrhoea also accompanies the above symptoms.

BRYONIA

Dry cough, fever, generalised body pain particularly in the chest wall.
Dryness is a feature of the lips and tongue.
Patient is prostrate and motionless.
Worse for the least heat and movement.

GELSEMIUM

In early stages with temperature, fatigue, weakness and general aching and soreness in the whole body, especially in the back area.
Patient is chilly, has a cough, face is flushed, eyes water and sneezing is frequent.

NUX VOM

Chilly.
Must be covered.
Body is burning hot, especially the face, but unable to move without feeling chilly.

*Tissue Salts*

CALC PHOS

Weakness and exhaustion.
Good for convalescing after 'flu.

FERR PHOS

Excellent generally where there is a high temperature and a quick pulse.

NAT SULPH

Excellent remedy as it removes excess fluids in the tissues.
Thick, ropy mucus.
Soreness and pain in left side of chest.
Hurts when coughing.

## Measles

Measles is a highly infectious virus. The symptoms usually appear approximately 10 - 15 days from contact. In the early stages, the symptoms are cold-like in nature with the rash appearing on the fourth day. The rash starts behind the ears and around the mouth and then spreads rapidly over the whole body. The spots are small, red blotches with a progressively yellowy tinge and can even be seen in the mouth. The rash lasts for roughly 4 days and can be accompanied by a sore throat and sensitive eyes. When caring for someone with measles, it is essential to keep them out of direct sunlight and in a shaded room to protect the eyes. As with any infection, particularly with a fever, it is important to keep up the liquid intake and prevent dehydration.

ACONITE
Cold-like symptoms in the initial stages. High fever, full pulse, dry cough, constipation, restlessness and thirst with anxiety.

BELLADONNA
Second stage. Temperature raised. Earache or headache.

BRYONIA
Tiresome, dry, painful cough. Headache with dry mouth and intense thirst for cold water. Sufferer is motionless. Irritable and worse for any movement or disturbance.

GELSEMIUM
High fever prominent with apathy and sluggishness. Watery nasal discharge which burns and inflames nose and upper lip. Eyelids drooping and heavy. Dry cough, sore chest.

PULSATILLA    Lack of thirst, restless and irritable.
Cough worse in evening.
Yellow catarrhal discharge from throat and nose.
Diarrhoea, intestinal and gastric upsets.
Rash.
Good for early stages.

*Tissue Salts*

FERR PHOS    Skin is hot and burning.
Throat painful and swollen.
Intolerance to any heat yet slightest cold draught is also intolerable.
Feeling of chilliness.

# Mumps

The cause of this illness is again a virus. The symptoms appear 14 - 21 days after contact when the glands begin to swell. The disease is infectious approximately 2 - 3 days before the symptoms appear until 7 days after the swelling goes. The symptoms include pain and swelling of the parotid glands in the neck. The pain is felt on opening and shutting the mouth and swallowing. It usually starts with one gland and may progress to other glands in the mouth and the neck. One gland settles down after 4 - 5 days and then the other gland may swell afterwards staying swollen for another 4 - 5 days. Mumps is uncomplicated in children but can be unpleasant in adults when the swelling can extend to testicles, breast and ovaries. The swelling of sexual organs is serious in men as it can affect fertility.

See the section on sore throats on page 77 for advice regarding hot and cold packs to relieve swelling and pain.

ACONITE          Fever, restlessness, thirst and pain in the
                 early acute stages.

BELLADONNA       Throbbing, burning skin, especially on the
                 face.
                 Glands swollen, hot, red, sensitive to
                 pressure and may be worse on the
                 right side.

MERCURIUS        Throat is raw and sore.
                 Testicles are swollen and hard.
                 Scrotum is shiny, red and itchy.

PULSATILLA       Swollen glands.
                 Inflamed or enlarged testicles or breasts.
                 Thick coating on the tongue, mouth dry but
                 with lack of thirst, even in fever.

RHUS TOX       Sore throat with swollen glands.
               Pain on swallowing.
               Cheekbones painful.
               General aches and pains and constant
               desire to change position.
               Swollen testicles.

*Tissue Salts*

FERR PHOS      Excellent generally, where there is a high
               temperature and a quick pulse.

# Tonsillitis

Tonsillitis is an unpleasant illness which recurs, particularly in childhood. The usual course of action is to surgically remove the tonsils. This is regrettable if there is another course of action as the tonsils contribute to the body's immune system. They are the guardians at the door of the throat!

The illness starts like a cold. The sufferer loses his or her appetite, feels shivery, feels tired and headachy and complains of a sore throat. Then small blisters of pus appear on the tonsils at the back of the throat. The glands in the neck can also swell and there is a sense of constriction in the throat. The temperature is raised, the tongue dry and coated and the face flushed. The breath can even be tainted. The infection lasts for approximately 10 days. Tonsillitis can be complicated by ear and chest infections and abscesses. It is an unpleasant and debilitating illness which affects adults as well as children.

Tonsillitis is an expression of lowered vitality. Health tonics like Floradix and Kindervitel are helpful, as is rest and a good nutritious diet. Gargling with salt and warm water and drinking red sage tea and fresh lemon with warm water and honey are also advised. If the infections return regularly, a visit to your homoeopath is recommended.

| | |
|---|---|
| ACONITE | Burning, smarting dryness.<br>Sudden onset.<br>Tingling sensation on swallowing. |
| BELLADONNA | Usually right sided.<br>Very acute attacks with redness and swelling of tonsil area.<br>Fever, neck stiff and inflamed.<br>Pain is severe. |
| HEPAR SULPH | Very infected area, with splinter-like pain on swallowing.<br>High temperature, shivering and abscess formation.<br>Sweaty. |

IGNATIA

Tonsils inflamed, hard and swollen.
White spots on tonsils.
Stitching pains extending to ear.
Painful glands.
Possibly has fever with red face, heat and no thirst.

LACHESIS

Infection starts on left side.
Tonsils are bluish and swollen.
Worse for swallowing liquids.
Better for solids.

MERCURIUS

Severe infection.
Yellow and ulcerated tonsils.
Bad breath, stinging throat with marked sweating and a temperature.
Metallic taste in mouth.

*Tissue Salts*

KALI MUR

White or grey spots on tonsils.
When swallowing is difficult.

NAT MUR

Clear mucus covers tonsils and much salivation.

SILICA

Helps heal septic tonsils.

## Whooping Cough

Whooping cough is a serious complaint in children but homoeopathic remedies can be very helpful in its treatment. Homoeopathy can also provide preventative (prophylactic) treatment for parents who do not want, or indeed cannot have, their child vaccinated. We suggest that you seek the advice of your practitioner in the prevention and treatment of this complaint.

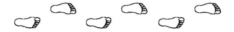

## Vaccinations

More and more children are being given vaccinations for infectious illnesses. Many parents accept the need for polio, diphtheria and tetanus but sometimes refuse the whooping cough vaccine and question the need for the combined vaccine for measles, mumps and rubella (known as MMR). The arguments for and against the vaccination of children are many and it is not within the scope of this book to analyse the debate. Some parents are now reluctant to allow their children to be vaccinated. If, as parents, you have made this choice, please make sure that your child at least has access to preventative homoeopathic treatment. Alternatively, if your child does become ill after receiving vaccinations, do not forget that a professional homoeopath can do much to relieve the distress this may cause.

# Chapter 17

# FIRST AID

A course in basic first aid is a must. Many lives have been saved by a good working knowledge of first aid procedures. Taking such a course is a responsible attitude to engender and may be the most important course you ever take in your life. Ill-informed help or no help at all can cause great damage to the unsuspecting victim.

## Burns & Scalds

If the burn is severe, it is important never to bandage or apply ointment or any other substance to the affected area. For minor burns and scalds, run the affected area under cold water for a few minutes. A very effective homoeopathic ointment for burns is available containing *Calendula* and *Cantharis*. Honey applied for minor burns is a good alternative.

ACONITE
: Shock.
Anxious, excited, nervous, feverish.
Acute, violent, painful situations.

APIS
: Shrieks very loudly with pain.
Stinging, smarting, lacerating pain with excessive swelling with red, rosy, shiny colour.

ARNICA
: Immediately, if there is shock or distress.

BELLADONNA
: Redness, throbbing, burning with much heat in affected area.

CANTHARIS       For the pain, particularly when there is
                formation of blisters and burning
                sensation, with the skin red and peeling.

HYPERICUM Ø     Externally in tincture.
                1 drop of tincture to 10 of water;
                applied locally, except in very severe cases.
                A useful antiseptic.

URTICA URENS    Burns and scalds with intense itching and
                blistering of the skin.

## Injuries

ARNICA ∅ — Externally in tincture.
1 drop of tincture to 10 of water;
applied locally provided the skin is not
broken.

ARNICA — Internally in pill form.
Immediately if there is shock or distress.
Concussion.
For bruising when there is pain and swelling.

CALENDULA ∅ — Externally in tincture.
1 drop of tincture to 10 of water;
applied locally when skin is broken, and
if the wounds are deep and lacerated and
give *Arnica* internally.

HYPERICUM — Internally in pill form.
To prevent sepsis.

HYPERICUM ∅ — Externally in tincture.
1 drop of tincture to 10 of water;
applied locally to injuries in areas rich in
sentient nerves, such as the ends of fingers
and toes.
Also for septic conditions.

LEDUM — Puncture wounds, e.g. from nails, needles etc..
Prevents infection if given immediately
after wounding.
Especially for black eyes.

RHUS TOX — Swollen, painful joints.
Better for hot applications and for
continued motion.

RUTA GRAV — For sprains of the ankle and wrists.
For sprains of tendons.
Bruised, sore and aching muscles.

SYMPHYTUM    All injuries to bones such as fractures or
             bruises.
             Helps to knit bones and promote healing.

## Surgical & Dental Operations

If you have a great dread of visiting the doctor or dentist, hypnosis can do much to relieve your suffering. It can also be a valuable tool for pain relief. A good practitioner of hypnotherapy can help you to overcome fears and anxiety. He or she can also teach you the technique of self-hypnosis which is simple and easy to use, even in the dentist's chair.

ACONITE — Helps allay fear before the event, especially with children.
After effects of surgical shock and injury.
Emotional and nervous tension.
Fear is very intense.
Fear accompanying most trivial ailments.

ARNICA — Should always be given before and after operations.
It will assist in clotting if bleeding persists.
Promotes rapid healing.
Prevents pus forming.

CALENDULA — Internally in pill form.
To promote healing.

CALENDULA ∅ — Externally in tincture.
1 drop of tincture to 10 of water;
applied directly on wound to promote healing after any operation.

## Bleeding

ARNICA              Always given first if bleeding follows injury.

IPECAC              Comes in gushes of bright red blood.
                    Good for nosebleed and uterine
                    haemorrhage, particularly if accompanied
                    by nausea.

PHOSPHORUS          Nose bleeds and small wounds which bleed
                    very easily.
                    Easily prostrated.
                    Wants sympathy.
                    Healed wounds which break out and bleed
                    again.

*Tissue Salts*

FERR PHOS           Bleeding internally or externally which
                    rapidly clots and is bright red.

## Stings & Bites

If stung by a honey bee, always scrape out the sting or flick it out with a fingernail. Do not pull it out because you will squeeze in more poison from the poison sacks and the sting is also barbed. If stung on the hand or foot, pour cold water in a bowl and add a tray of ice cubes plus 4 teaspoons of baking soda. Stir and place the stung area in the mixture until relieved.

For those who have an allergic reaction to bee or wasp stings, *Apis* taken one pill a day for three days at the beginning of spring is a sensible precautionary measure. This will, in many cases, reduce the potentially painful and sometimes dangerous effects of being stung.

APIS

Stings and bites, when there is much red, hot swelling with agonising pain.
Especially good for insect stings and bites.

LEDUM

For bites from small animals or insects.
Puncture wounds.
Prevents infection if given immediately after wounding.

# Chapter 18

# WHEN TO SEEK
# MEDICAL ADVICE AND TREATMENT?

This book is primarily written to help prescribe homoeopathic remedies for simple first aid situations and common ailments. It is not a guide to the treatment of serious complaints or a substitute for your qualified practitioner. Furthermore, there are instances which warrant the calling out of a medical practitioner, especially in infants, and we are at pains to stress that any instances which cause concern should be dealt with by professionals.

It is up to the individual whether he or she seeks orthodox medical help or consults a homoeopath or another natural medicine practitioner. In the case of serious accident and injuries your local casualty department is the first place to go. Natural medicine can aid recovery but it cannot stitch wounds and set bones! Remember orthodox diagnosis is available to everyone and it can put your mind at rest. If you prefer a natural alternative to a prescribed drug, discuss this with the medical practitioner, many are willing to co-operate.

Please seek medical advice in the event of conditions as listed in this chapter.

## Head

Sharp or hard blows to the head, especially if they cause
even momentary unconsciousness;
persistent headaches when it is unusual;
recurrent or chronic dizzy spells;
bulging, tense fontanelle, accompanied possibly by fever
and rash in a baby;
ear complaints, especially when there is pain and fever -
seek medical advice within 24 hours, especially with
children;
eye complaints such as pain, wounds, and visual changes;
nasal obstructions;
swellings on the external neck or glands;
convulsions;
severe muscle weakness or loss of feeling.

## Chest

Breathing difficulties, especially if the ribs stand out with
effort;
waking up due to breathing difficulties at night;
a chronic or persistent cough, especially with the spitting
of blood;
asthma, if it is getting progressively worse;
listlessness with rapid shallow breathing;
wheezing due to a history of weak heart or lung problems;
pains through the chest (more often heart than
lung problems);
heart palpitations;
shortness of breath on mild exertion.

## Abdomen

For diarrhoea and vomiting, make sure the patient does not become dehydrated. Encourage sips of water little and often. Seek medical advice if symptoms persist for more than 24 hours or when there is a stomach pain which becomes worse or persistent vomiting, with weakness, listlessness and floppy head and limbs, lack of appetite, especially in a baby.

Also be wary of:
any sign of intestinal obstruction accompanied by sharp pain, vomiting, abdominal swelling and constipation;
any swelling in the abdomen which occurs in a short time;
pains in the top right hand side of the pelvis;
any lump with or without swelling and distention;
any abdominal complaint in pregnant women, especially if in one particular place;
radiating pains to the groin, suggesting kidney problems;
any changes in the bowel habit, especially for those over 50;
any bleeding whatsoever from the rectum;
black or bloody stools.

## Sexual & Urinary Organs

Any painful lump in the groin or testicles;
excessively frequent urination;
constant thirst and frequency of urination.

# Fevers

Help to keep down fevers by removing clothes and sponging with tepid water. Do not, however, allow the patient to get cold and excessively shivery.

Be wary of:
prolonged high temperatures, especially in babies;
lying with the head drawn back, accompanied possibly by high fever and rash;
any twitching or sign of a fit.

# General Symptoms & States

Excessive weakness at any age;
any lump or enlarged gland anywhere, especially in the breast, armpit, groin, and neck;
continuous loss of weight even though eating well;
backache if severe and continued;
red sputum.

# Accidents

Any burn which is too severe for self-treatment;
large wounds;
broken bones.

Common sense will usually help you to decide whether a visit to casualty is indicated or a visit to your practitioner. Whatever the case, do not delay if you are concerned. Many symptoms turn out to be minor and lumps and bumps appear all over the body as we age, although it is not worth ignoring them or waiting for any of the above conditions to pass. Proper medical diagnosis and treatment can allay many fears and as we have said before natural medicine can work very well with its orthodox partner.

# Appendix 1

# MATERIA MEDICA
# OF
# REMEDIES USED IN THIS BOOK

This mini *materia medica* gives an overall 'picture' of the primary symptoms characteristic of each remedy. It can be used to help confirm the choice of remedy you have made from the main prescribing section of this book (Section Two).

# Materia Medica

ACONITE *(Aconitum Napellus)* - Monk's Hood

Full of fears and tosses about as if in agony.
Restlessness and inconsolable anxiety.
Heat, with inclination to uncover oneself.
Local numbness or tingling.
Complaints from exposure to dry, cold winds and draughts.
Desire for bitter drinks.
Worse for lying on the left or affected side;
when rising from bed;
in the evening and at night; in a warm room.
Better for open air.

AESCULUS *(Aesculus Hippocastanum)* - Horse Chestnut

Haemorrhoids: purple, painful, external, with backache.
Stools followed by fullness of rectum and intense pain in anus for hours.
Knife-like pains shoot up the rectum.
Large haemorrhoids which block up the rectum without much loss of blood.
Despondent, gloomy, very irritable, loses temper easily and gains control slowly.
Chill better for heat.
Worse for inhaling cold air; motion; walking; stooping; washing in water; in winter.
Better in summer.

## ALLIUM CEPA - Red Onion

Headache with cold in the head.
Streaming eyes and nose from odour of peaches or
flowers.
Copious watery discharge from the nose with tears.
Frequent and violent sneezing, particularly on
entering a warm room.
Cough compels sufferer to grasp the larynx;
seems as if cough would tear it.
Worse in the evening and in a warm room.
Better in cold room and open air.


## ALUMINA - Oxide of Aluminium

Attacks of depression.
Loss of memory; time passes slowly.
Abnormal appetite: wants starch, chalk, charcoal,
coffee or tea, acids, indigestible things.
Potatoes disagree.
Constipation: no desire for and no ability to pass
stools until there is a large accumulation.
The stools may be dry, hard and knotty, like sheep
dung, or soft.
Inactivity of the rectum: even a small stool requires
great straining.
Worse for cold air; sitting; eating soups;
during winter; on alternate days; at new and full
moon.
Better for mild summer weather; warm drinks;
wet weather; while eating.

## ANT TART *(Antimonium Tartaricum)*
### Tartrate of Antimony and Potash

Great debility and weakness.

The child wants to be carried but does not wish to be touched.

Great sleepiness or irresistible inclination to sleep with nearly all complaints.

Respiratory troubles with great accumulation of mucus, but with difficulty in expectoration.

Prostration with great drowsiness and cold sweat.

Worse for damp, cold weather; lying down at night; change of weather in spring; in a warm room.

Better for cold, open air; sitting upright; expectoration; lying on the right side.


## APIS *(Apis Mellifica)* - Honey Bee

Burning and stinging pains.

Sensation of not being able to breathe.

Stinging and throbbing; very sensitive to touch.

Intermittent fever: chill worse around 3 p.m. and always accompanied by thirst.

Lack of thirst in most complaints.

Anxiety with tearful restlessness.

Impaired memory and absent-mindedness in elderly persons.

Watery swellings.

Worse in a warm room and from external heat; after sleeping.

Better for open air; cold bathing; uncovering; sitting erect.

## ARG NIT *(Argentum Nitricum)* - Silver Nitrate

Impulsive, time seems too short.
Wants to do things in a hurry.
Must walk fast; is always hurried.
Apprehension before events, often accompanied
by diarrhoea.
Belching accompanies most gastric ailments.
Sensation of a splinter, especially in the throat.
Sugar craving; child is fond of it, but diarrhoea
results from eating it.
Worse for cold food; cold air; eating sugar or
ice cream; thinking intently.
Better for open air; wind blowing in face; bathing
in cold water.

## ARNICA *(Arnica Montana)* - Leopard's Bane

Sore, lame, bruised feeling all through the body,
as if beaten.
Traumatic affections of muscles.
Bad effects from mechanical injuries (falls and
bruises etc.).
Says he or she is well, when very sick.
Bruised, sore feeling all over; bed feels too hard.
Belching: offensive odour like rotten eggs.
Worse for rest; lying down; wine.
Better for motion.

ARS ALB *(Arsenicum Album)* - Arsenic

Anxiety and restlessness very highly marked.
Fear, fright and worry.
Excessive exhaustion from slightest exertion.
Watery head cold; discharge causes burning or
smarting of nostrils as if sore.
Burning pains.
Great fastidiousness.
Great prostration.
Fear of the dark.
Worse from 1 to 2 p.m. or 12 to 2 a.m..
Better for heat in all complaints except headache,
which is temporarily relieved by cold bathing.

BELLADONNA - Deadly Nightshade

Lively and entertaining people when well but
violent and often delirious when sick.
Furious delirium with a wild look; wishes to strike,
bite or quarrel; face flushed and eyes red.
Almost constantly moaning.
Over-sensitivity of all the senses.
Sleepiness, but cannot sleep.
Pupils dilated.
Aversion to light.
Sudden onset of inflammation.
Ailments predominantly right-sided.
Worse for touch; motion; noise; drafts;
looking at bright, shining objects; after 3 p.m.;
while drinking; uncovering the head; summer sun;
lying down.
Better for rest; standing or sitting erect;
being in a warm room.

## BRYONIA *(Bryonia Alba)* - Wild Hop

An irritable mood and inclined to be angry.
The child dislikes to be carried or to be raised.
Headache as if the head would split open: greatly
aggravated by motion, opening the eyes, or stooping;
relieved by pressure and closing the eyes.
Sharp, stitching pains.
Cannot sit up from nausea and faintness.
Great thirst for large volume of liquid, but at long
intervals.
Pressure in the pit of the stomach, as if there was a
stone in it, relieved by belching.
Worse for slightest motion of any kind; exertion;
touch; sitting up; warmth; warm food.
Better for mental and physical rest; pressure; cold;
lying, especially on painful side; eating cold things.

## CALC CARB *(Calcarea Carbonica)* - Carbonate of Calcium

Often suitable for difficulty or delay in cutting or
growing of teeth in children.
For children that have a tendency to grow fat.
Anxiety of mind.
Shortness of breath, especially on going upstairs.
Painful swelling of the glands.
Vomiting of sour substances.
Great longing for eggs.
White chalk-like stools.
Easy sweating; mainly of the head.
Deficient circulation: coldness and clamminess of
single parts especially the legs, feet and hands.
Worse for mental exertion; eating;
cold and wet weather; fasting; cold water;
washing; on awakening; in the morning;
in the evening; after midnight; during full moon.
Better for rubbing; drawing the limbs up;
lying on back; the dark; dry weather;
lying on the painful side; when constipated.

## CALENDULA *(Calendula Officinalis)* - Marigold

External wounds and lacerations, with or without
loss of substance.
Ulcers: irritable; inflamed; varicose;
painful as if beaten; excessive secretion of pus.
Particularly useful in the dressing of torn or cut
wounds, the parts being kept wet constantly with
a weak solution.
Worse for damp weather; in the evening.
Better for warmth.

## CANTHARIS - Spanish Fly

Intense irritation, both mental and physical.
Violent cutting, burning pains.
Retention of urine with spasmodic pain in the
bladder.
Constant desire to urinate, passing but a few drops
at a time, sometimes mixed with blood.
Drinking even small quantities of water increases
pain in the bladder.
Intense inflammation of the skin with the
formation of blisters.
Worse for drinking coffee; the sight of water and
bright objects; touch or approach; at night;
while drinking; before, during and after passing
urine.
Better for rubbing; lying down quietly on the back.

## CAUSTICUM - Hahnemann's Tinctura Acris Sine Kali

Melancholy mood.
General respiratory and urinary problems.
Morning hoarseness.
Cough accompanied by a spurt of urine.
Involuntary emission of urine when sneezing,
blowing the nose or walking.
Stools pass better when standing.
Worse for clear fine weather; coming from the
open air into a warm room; cold air;
getting wet or bathing.
Better for damp, wet weather; warm air.

## CHAMOMILLA - German Chamomile

The child who wants to be carried and is then more
quiet.
Excessively fretful child; is only quiet if carried up
and down the room all the time.
Ailments caused by anger.
Great sense of debility out of all proportion to the
seriousness of the disease.
Pain that seems unendurable, drives the sufferer to
despair.
Worse for heat; anger; open air; belching;
in the wind; in the evening before midnight.
Better for being carried; fasting; warm, wet weather.

CHINA *(Cinchona Officinalis)* - Peruvian Bark

> Regularly recurring symptoms, particularly every other day.
> Intense throbbing headache, after excessive haemorrhage.
> Debilitation from loss of vital fluids, especially haemorrhages, excessive lactation, diarrhoea or suppurations.
> Worse for slightest touch; draughts; mental or physical exertion.
> Better for hard pressure; bending double.


COCCULUS *(Cocculus Indicus)* - Indian Cockle

> Sensation of emptiness or hollowness.
> Cannot bear the slightest contradiction.
> Time passes too quickly.
> Complaints from loss of sleep.
> Seasickness.
> Swimming and giddiness with nausea.
> Aversion to food.
> Loathing of food even when merely looking at it.
> Desire for cold drinks, especially beer.
> Worse for eating; drinking; smoking; talking; motion of ship; rising from sitting position during pregnancy.
> Better in a warm room; when lying quiet.

## COFFEA *(Coffea Cruda)* - Coffee

Excited and over-sensitive.
Great sensitivity to pain; driven to despair with weeping.
Sleeplessness on account of excessive excitability of the mind and of the body.
Headache: one-sided, as from nail driven into the brain.
Worse for excessive joy; excess of wine; cold, open air; narcotics.
Better for cold water; lying down.

## COLOCYNTH *(Colocynthis)* - Bitter Cucumber

A violent, agonising abdominal colic, relieved by bending double and by pressing something hard into the abdomen.
Anger with indignation.
Colic, better from lying on the abdomen.
Sciatica, cramp in hip.
Worse for anger; cheese; in the evening; after eating.
Better for doubling up; hard pressure.

## DROSERA - Sundew

Whooping cough, with bleeding from the nose and mouth with a nightly aggravation.
Constant tickly cough in children, begins as soon as the head touches the pillow at night.
Constriction of the chest.
Worse for heat; warmth; drinking; singing; laughing; weeping; lying down; during rest; after midnight and early morning.
Better for motion; cold air; sitting up in bed; remaining quiet.

## EUPHRASIA - Eyebright

Catarrhal infections of the mucous membranes, especially of the eyes and nose.
Eyes water all the time and are gummed-up in the morning; margins of lids red, swollen, burning.
Aversion to light.
Whooping cough: watering eyes during cough; cough in daytime.
Worse for being in bed; being indoors; warmth; after exposure to south wind; in the evening.
Better for being in the dark; open air; wiping the eyes.

## GELSEMIUM - Yellow Jasmine

For children and young people, especially women
of a nervous, emotional temperament.
Confusion of the mind.
Fear of falling; the child grasps the cot or seizes the
adult.
The anticipation of any unusual ordeal;
preparing for an outing or meeting brings on
diarrhoea.
Headache, principally in the back of head;
better for reclining the head and shoulders on a
high pillow.
Great heaviness of the eyelids; cannot keep them
open.
Lack of muscular co-ordination; confused;
muscles refuse to obey the will.
First stages of a fever.
Worse for damp weather; before a thunder-storm;
excitement; bad news; smoking; when thinking of
ailments; when spoken to of a loss.
Better for profuse urination; remaining quiet.

## GLONOINE - Nitroglycerine

Confusion; loss of orientation; well-known streets
seem strange.
Head feels enormously large.
Headache from below upwards; brain as if moving
in waves.
Headache from recent exposure to sun.
Headache instead of periods.
Afraid to shake the head; it increases the ache and
seems as though the head would drop in pieces.
Worse for sun; overheating; stooping; ascending;
having hair cut.
Better for cold air; pressure.

## GRAPHITES - Black Lead

Women inclined to obesity, who suffer from habitual constipation, with a history of delayed menstruation.
Great sadness and despondency with inclination to weep, especially at hearing music.
Unhealthy skin.
Itching eruptions with oozing of corrosive, clear and sticky fluid.
Skin dry, nails become hard, thick and brittle.
Glandular swellings.
Constipation; large, difficult, knotty stools.
Very weak and prostrated during menses.
Ear troubles; hears better in a background noise.
Worse for cold; draughts; during and after menses; at night; daylight; suppressed menstruation.
Better for open air; hot drinks, especially milk; when surrounded by noise.

## HAMAMELIS *(Hamamelis Virginica)* - Witch Hazel

Much weariness, gets tired easily.
Hammering headache.
Nose bleeds.
Haemorrhoids bleed very profusely with sensation of soreness, weight and burning in the rectum; they protrude, and anus feels sore as if raw.
Varicose veins: hard, knotty, swollen and painful.
Injuries from falls.
Bruised soreness.
Worse for pressure; exposure to cold air; touch; motion.
Better for rest; lying quietly.

## HEPAR SULP *(Hepar Sulphuris Calcareum)*
### Hahnemann's Calcium Sulphide

Great sensitiveness of the affected parts to touch.
Fainting in the evening from trifling pains.
Over-sensitive, physically and mentally;
irritated by the slightest thing.
Hasty speech and drinking.
Clay coloured stools.
Unhealthy skin; every little wound gathers pus.
Profuse discharges; smell like old cheese.
Sweats profusely day and night, without relief.
Sharp splinter-like pains in the throat.
Worse for cold, dry air; uncovering; touch;
lying on the painful part; draughts; at night;
in winter.
Better for warmth; wrapping up, especially the head.

## HYPERICUM - St. John's Wort

Injuries from treading on nails, needles, pins,
splinters, or from rat bites; prevents lock-jaw.
Injuries to parts rich in sentient nerves, especially
in fingers, toes, and matrices of nails.
Nervous depression following wounds or surgical
operations.
Bad effects from falls or blows upon the head,
or concussion of the spine.
Intolerably violent pains along the nerves.
Worse for motion; touch; shock; at night.
Better for lying quietly; rubbing.

# IGNATIA - St. Ignatius Bean

Women of a sensitive, easily excited nature.
Bad effects from fright, sorrow, offences and
unfortunate love affairs.
Spasmodic and hysterical complaints.
Rapid change of mood; jesting and laughter
changing to sadness and tears.
Moodiness.
Full of silent grief; sits down and sighs.
Weak empty feeling in the pit of the stomach, not
relieved by eating.
Worse for open air; cold air; tobacco; coffee;
touch; stooping; walking; standing; yawning.
Better for change of position; lying on affected part;
urination; swallowing; eating; sour things;
warmth.

# IPECAC *(Ipecacuanha)* - Ipecac

When gastric symptoms predominate.
Dry, spasmodic cough, ending in choking and
gagging.
Tongue clean in spite of internal disorder.
All diseases with constant and continual nausea.
Violent and persistent nausea, not relieved by
vomiting.
Haemorrhages of bright red, gushing blood.
Respiratory complaints.
Worse for warmth; overeating; damp;
slightest motion; rich foods.
Better for open air; rest; pressure; closing eyes;
cold drinks.

## LACHESIS - Bushmaster or Surukuku Snake Venom

Thin and emaciated rather than fleshy persons.
Those who have been changed, both mentally and physically, by their illness.
Women who have not recovered from the change of life and have never felt well since that time.
Very talkative.
Suspicious and jealous.
All problems with sleep: sleepiness but cannot sleep; sleep disturbed by frightful dreams etc..
Left side principally affected; diseases begin on the left side and move to the right side, i.e. left ovary, testicle, chest etc..
Tonsillitis or diphtheria, worse on the left side; choking when swallowing, or pain from the throat into the ear; neck very sensitive to touch; aggravation after sleep.
Great sensitiveness to touch, pressure and constriction; even of clothing, especially around the throat and abdomen.
Pressing or bursting in the temples.
Bluish discharges.
Worse for motion; touch; constriction; pressure; stooping; lying; after sleeping; heat; in summer; swallowing; hot drinks.
Better for open air; onset of a discharge; cold drinks; hard pressure.

LEDUM - Marsh Tea

Always feels cold and chilly, yet averse to external warmth.
Insect stings and bites, especially mosquitoes.
Puncture wounds.
Rheumatic and arthritic complaints; begins below and travels upward.
Affected parts become purple and puffy.
Haemorrhages of bright, frothy blood.
Worse for motion; warmth of bed and bed covering; alcohol; while walking; at night.
Better for putting feet in ice-water; cool air; while resting.


LYCOPODIUM *(Lycopodium Clavatum)* - Club Moss

Ailments that develop gradually.
For persons who are intellectually keen but physically weak.
Lacks self-confidence.
Baby cries all day and sleeps all night.
Snuffles: the child wakes from sleep rubbing nose.
Afraid to be left alone.
Very sensitive, even cries when thanked.
Irritable: peevish and cross on waking; kicks and screams; easily angered; cannot endure opposition or contradiction; seeks disputes.
Great flatulence.
Hungry, but full up after a few mouthfuls.
Complaints that are right-sided or that travel from right to left.
Worse for pressure of clothes; warmth; eating; from 4 p.m. to 8 p.m..
Better for warm drinks; belching; motion; urinating.

MERCURIUS *(Mercurius Solubilis)* - Black Oxide of Mercury

Deficient memory and will power.
Weakness and weariness in all the limbs, with
pronounced tremor.
Glands enlarged.
Conditions with pus formations.
Profuse salivation with metallic taste.
Tongue swollen and flabby, showing teeth imprints.
Moist tongue, but with great thirst.
Ulcerations, especially around the mouth and throat.
Worse for sweating; lying on the right side;
warmth of bed; draughts to the head; heat and cold;
during and after urination; at night.
Better for moderate temperatures; rest.


NAT MUR *(Natrum Muriaticum)* - Common Salt

The most weakness is felt in the morning in bed.
Great emaciation.
Splitting headache.
Consolation aggravates.
Bad effects of using too much salt.
Great dryness of the mucous membranes from the
lips to the anus; lips dry and cracked, especially in
the middle; anus dry, cracked, fissured.
Worse for lying down, especially on the left side;
noise; heat; heat of the sun; hot weather;
mental exertion; at sea-shore; in the morning from
10 a.m. to 11 a.m.; at night.
Better for sweating; open air; cold bathing;
lying on the right side; pressure; from tight clothing;
while fasting.

## NIT AC *(Nitricum Acidum)* - Nitric Acid

Problems concerning the mucous outlets of the
body where the skin and mucous membrane join,
i.e. the mouth, nose, rectum, anus, urethra and vagina.
Ailments from the change of weather.
Ailments are predominantly right-sided.
Great debility and trembling, especially in the
morning.
Offensive odour of breath.
Cracking in the joints on motion.
Cutting or pricking pain, as from splinters,
especially on touching the part.
Sensation of a band around the head.
Urine dark brown and strong smelling.
Ulcerations.
Worse for milk; loss of sleep; changing weather;
touch; at night.
Better for car travel; mild weather; steady pressure.


## NUX VOM *(Nux Vomica)* - Poison Nut

Angry and impatient; cannot stand pain.
Quarrelsome, irritable and irascible.
Mental and physical hypersensitivity.
Drowsiness during evening, wakeful at
3 a.m. to 4 a.m..
Digestive disorders.
Hunger, yet no desire for food.
Nausea and vomiting after eating.
Constipation; frequent but ineffective desire to
defecate..
Worse for cold; uncovering; high living; coffea;
condiments; liquor; drugs; purgatives;
mental exertion; pressure of clothes at waist;
in early morning.
Better for discharges; wrapping head; milk;
moist air; lying on sides; resting.

## PETROLEUM - Crude Rock-Oil

Symptoms appear and disappear rapidly.
General travel sickness.
Vertigo in the back of the head, like seasickness.
Irritable, quarrelsome disposition.
Cold feeling in the abdomen.
Diarrhoea, only in the daytime.
Gastric complaints, better by constant eating.
Dry, rough and cracked skin, especially tips of fingers.
Skin symptoms are worse in the winter, better in summer; and, if suppressed, cause diarrhoea.
Worse for travel motion; thunderstorms; touch;
Better for warm air; dry weather; lying with the head high.

## PHOSPHORUS - Phosphorus

For tall, nervous, weak and delicate persons.
Burning heat running up the back and between the shoulders.
Emaciation.
Great sensitiveness of the senses and giddiness.
Anxious and fearful before and during a thunder-storm.
Fear of being alone.
Apathetic: unwilling to talk; answers slowly; moves sluggishly.
Ravenous hunger during fever.
Weary of life, full of fears.
Tightness in chest.
Empty feeling in abdomen.
Craves salt.
Small wounds bleed much.
Worse for lying on the left side; cold; salt; mental fatigue; in the morning and evening; sudden change of weather; during a thunder-storm.
Better for eating; sleep; cold food and water.

## PHYTOLACCA - Poke Root

Indifference to life.
Aching, bruised soreness in all the muscles.
Rheumatic pains, shooting like electric shocks;
worse for motion.
Throat complaints; burning and dryness.
Mammary disorders; painful breasts, full, hard
and stoney.
Right-sided pains and complaints.
Worse for damp, cold weather; motion;
swallowing hot drinks; when rising from bed.
Better for lying on abdomen; rest; dry weather.

## PULSATILLA - Wind Flower

Timid and fearful, extremely mild and gentle and
sometimes silent and melancholic.
Weeps very easily at everything, whether joyful or
sorrowful.
Easily moved to laughter and tears.
Secretions from all the mucous membranes are
thick, bland and yellowish-green.
Nothing tastes good.
Absence of thirst with nearly all complaints.
Repugnance to food.
Chilly, yet averse to heat.
Symptoms ever-changing; no two chills, no two
stools, no two attacks alike: very well one hour,
very miserable the next - apparently contradictory.
Catarrh; greenish-yellow, thick and bland.
Gastric complaints from eating rich foods, fat, pork.
Menstrual disorders; delayed and irregular.
Worse for warmth; in a warm, closed room;
getting feet wet; in evening; rest; motion; eating;
rich foods; puberty; pregnancy; before menses.
Better for cold , fresh, open air; gentle motion;
erect posture; a good cry; rubbing;
lying with head high.

## RHUS TOX *(Rhus Toxicodendron)* - Poison Ivy

Great sadness and apprehension, with inclination
to weep.
Headache relieved by motion.
Pains in the back which compel constant
movement in bed.
Rheumatic complaint.
The pain and stiffness is worse on commencing
movement, but continued motion relieves.
Sciatica.
Influenza, with aching in the bones, sneezing and
coughing; dry cough; bronchial coughs in old
people.
Red, dry, cracked coated tongue with triangular
red tip.
Complaints which are generally right-sided.
Skin eruptions; surface raw, thick crusts, oozing
and offensive.
Worse for exposure to wet, cold air and draughts;
uncovering; beginning of motion; rest; before
storms; after midnight.
Better for continued motion; heat; hot bath;
warm wrapping; rubbing; change of position.

## RUTA GRAV *(Ruta Graveoleus)* - Rue

Bruises and other mechanical injuries of bones and the membranes surrounding the bones.
Soreness and lameness as from a sprain or bruise.
Wrists feel as if sprained and stiff; worse in cold, wet weather.
Eyes ache and feel strained; from fine sewing or reading, particularly by poor light.
Backache, relieved by lying on the back.
Worse for over-exertion; eye strain; cold air; sitting; pressure; stooping.
Better for lying on back; warmth; motion; rubbing; scratching.

## SEPIA - Inky Juice of Cuttlefish

Symptoms relieved from violent exertions, but reappear when sitting quietly in the morning and evening.
Weakness and faintness.
Dullness and indifference, especially in the family; also lack of interest in occupation.
Melancholy; worse for consolation and company.
Sudden prostration.
Sinking feeling in stomach, not relieved by eating.
Great pressure and bearing down in pelvic region.
Constipation during pregnancy.
Suppressed menstruation.
Ailments during pregnancy.
Flushes of heat and perspiration at the menopause.
Worse for cold air; in pregnancy; before menses; during menopause; in the morning and evening; after sleep; kneeling.
Better for violent motion; warmth of bed; pressure; crossing or drawing limbs up; open air.

## SILICA *(Silicea)* - Pure Flint

Anxious, yielding, timid; desires consolation.
Lacks confidence.
Want of heat; always chilly, even when exercising.
Catches cold easily especially when feet and head
are uncovered.
Feet sweat, with rawness or bad odour between
the toes.
Daily headache beginning in the neck.
Great perspiration in children, characteristically
about the head.
Headaches; worse from noise, mental exertion,
jarring; better for binding the head tightly or
wrapping the head warmly.
Constipation from weakness of rectum.
Ingrowing toenails.
Suppurations; remedy matures boils.
Worse for cold; during menses; at new moon;
uncovering, especially the head; from lying down;
after vaccination; draughts; pressure; motion;
open air; at night.
Better for warmth, especially from wrapping up
the head; in a warm room; in summer.

## SULPHUR - Sublimated Sulphur

Great weakness; sallow, pale and yellow face; with marked anaemia.
Mental and physical inertia; selfish and self-important.
Loss of vital strength.
Complaints that constantly relapse.
Chronic constitutional grumbler.
Untidy and dirty; intolerant of bathing.
Cannot wait for lunch.
Drinks much, eats little.
Burning sensation everywhere; puts the feet out of bed at night to keep them cool.
Itching worse from the heat of the bed.
Redness of orifices.
Diarrhoea; worse in the morning driving sufferer out of bed.
All the eruptions are greatly aggravated by washing and by being wet; wetting produces burning.
Standing is the most disagreeable position.
Worse for bathing; milk; atmospheric changes; warmth of bed or from over-exertion; talking; at 11 a.m.; during menopause; standing.
Better for open air; motion; walking; drawing up the affected limbs; sweating; dry, warm weather; lying on the right side.

## SYMPHYTUM - Comfrey

Injuries to the eye; great pain in the eye-ball.
Fractures.
Broken bones where the bones refuse to knit.
Worse for touch; motion; pressure; after mechanical injury.
Better for warmth.

## THUJA *(Thuja Occidentalis)* - Arbor Vitae

Bad effects following vaccination; never well since.
Always in a hurry, talks hurriedly, moves hurriedly, and is excitable.
Shivering through and through, from slightest uncovering of the body in warm air.
Sweats only on uncovered parts.
Chronic headaches with mental confusion; pain as if pierced by a nail.
Cough by day only.
Catarrh; with thick, green mucous discharge.
Diarrhoea; sudden, gurgling and explosive.
Warts, figwarts, polypi.
Worse for heat of the bed; cold, damp air; stretching; excessive tea drinking; narcotics; tobacco; spirituous liquors; at night; at 3 a.m. and 3p.m.; after vaccination.
Better for warm wrapping; sneezing; drawing up the limbs; crossing legs; touch.

## URTICA URENS - Stinging Nettle

General stinging, burning pains.
Urticaria (nettlerash), with intolerable itching and burning.
Urticaria alternating with rheumatism (alternating with asthma).
Urticaria; the skin becomes elevated, with a white central spot and a red areola, with stinging and burning relieved by rubbing.
Burns.
Haemorrhages.
Worse for cool, moist air; cool bathing; eating shell-fish; rising up; touch; after childbirth; during rheumatism; at night.
Better for rubbing; lying down.

# Appendix 2

# DIRECTORY OF SERVICES

# The
## Hyden House
# Holistic Emporium

Hyden House is a company run by a group of people devoted to holistic approaches and values. This includes the way in which we run our business, grow our food, recycle our outputs and our impact on our environment, both locally and globally.

With this mind, we have put together the *Holistic Emporium* catalogue of products which we feel are informative, useful and that can be difficult to acquire in the shops. The catalogue has a wide variety of products which include books, homoeopathic first aid kits, remedies and ointments for the beginner and the established prescriber, the finest, pure aromatherapy oils, waterless cookware, worm bins for making the champagne of composts, Hopi ear candles, banana chairs, Bach Flower remedies, Royal Jelly in vials and special invigorating teas. This is just a small selection of our unusual range of goods.

We also specialise in products for practitioners. Please tell us whether you wish to receive our additional list for natural medicine professionals.

If you would like to receive a free copy of the *Holistic Emporium* catalogue please telephone, fax or write to:

Hyden House Limited
Little Hyden Lane
Clanfield
Hampshire
PO8 0RU
Tel 0705 596500
Fax 0705 595834

# *Healthy* **Business**

## The Natural Practitioner's Guide To Success

by
Madeleine Harland & Glen Finn

*Healthy Business* is a book for everyone considering a rewarding career in natural medicine as well as for those who are already in practise. It is the first book to clearly detail how to establish and run a successful natural health practice and to investigate the gritty reality of managing clinics as businesses. A troubleshooting guide, it offers practical advice which demystifies every area of marketing and management and is tailor-made for the natural health practitioner.

*Healthy Business* is highly inspirational and holistic in quality, harmoniously marrying both pragmatism and enthusiasm. It is about dealing with *real* situations and *real* people and not just the bank balance.

Short-listed for Lambert's 1990 Book of the Year award, this unique book has also been widely acclaimed as invaluable by colleges, societies, and experienced practitioners.

### No Nonsense Money Back Guarantee

Whether you are starting a career in natural medicine or already successfully in practice, we personally guarantee that you will find something of value in *Healthy Business* or we will give you your money back.

*Healthy Business*
*The Natural Practitioner's Guide to Success*
160pp, Hardback, Price £12.95 + £1.00 p&p

Available by return from:
Hyden House Limited
Little Hyden Lane, Clanfield, Hampshire PO8 0RU
Telephone 0705 596500 Fax 0705 595834

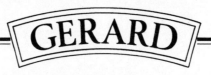
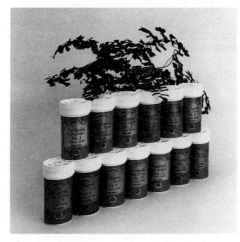

By Appointment to
Her Majesty The Queen
Chemists

By Appointment to
Her Majesty Queen Elizabeth
The Queen Mother
Chemists

By Appointment to
H.R.H. The Prince of Wales
Suppliers of Homoeopathic
Medicines

# *Ainsworths*
## HOMOEOPATHIC
## PHARMACY

*'REMEDIES BY RETURN'*

**38 New Cavendish Street, London W1M 7LH**
Prescriptions: 071-935 5330   Fax: 071-486 4313
Answer Phone: 071-487 5253

*ORDERS ACCOUNTS BOOKS*
40-44 High Street, Caterham, Surrey CR3 5UB
Tel. Caterham (0883) 340332   Fax. (0883) 344602

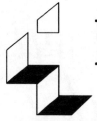

# THE BRITISH INSTITUTE
# OF
# HOMOEOPATHY

Supervised, Open University style, home study courses.

Introductory Course for beginners.

Advanced Course leading to award of
the Institute Diploma, DIHom.

*For free Prospectus, write: -*
The Registrar
The British Institute of Homoeopathy
427 Great West Road
Hounslow
Middlesex TW5 0BY
Tel: 081-577 7781

---

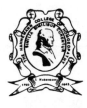

# THE HAHNEMANN COLLEGE
# OF
# HOMOEOPATHY
## (est. 1980)

Three year part time Diploma Course for beginners and
paramedics in Classical Homoeopathy.

Beginners preparatory course begins from May to July.

*For College prospectus, write to:*

The Secretary
243 The Broadway
Southall
Middlesex UB1 1NF
Tel: 081-843 9220/081-577 7781
Fax: 081-843 9220

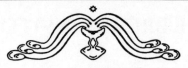

# *The School of Homoeopathy*

## CORRESPONDENCE FOUNDATION COURSE & PRACTITIONER DIPLOMA COURSE

Interested in learning more about homoeopathy? Join our one year Correspondence Course (Open University style) to thoroughly learn the basic principles and to study many useful remedies. Continue on to our part-time course to gain your practitioner's diploma, followed by a post-graduate year of supervised practice, leading to Registered Membership of the Society of Homoeopaths.

*For full details of these comprehensive courses, please send an A5 sae to The Administrator (B) at:*

**The School of Homoeopathy, Yondercott House Uffculme, Devon EX15 3DR**

 THE COLLEGE OF HOMŒOPATHY

REGENT'S COLLEGE • INNER CIRCLE • REGENT'S PARK • LONDON NW1 4NS

Established 1978

**Could you see yourself as a professional homœopath?** Running your own independent practice, treating the people of your choice with the values and care which you believe they deserve?

If you are 21 years or over, serious in your interest, and want to train with an established and reputable college, the College of Homœopathy has trained more than half the professional homœopaths in the UK and offers suitable candidates the opportunity to enrol on Britain's most successful course of homœopathic education to practitioner standard.
Part-time and Full-time programmes

**Contact us today on 071 487 7416 for more information.**

# THE LONDON COLLEGE
## OF
## CLASSICAL HOMOEOPATHY

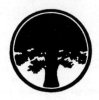

**Full Time and Part Time Professional Training Courses**
**in**
**CLASSICAL HOMOEOPATHY**

Also **Introductory/Foundation** and **Post Graduate Courses.**

*For details and prospectus please send £1.00 and A5 s.a.e. to:*
The Registrar (BH),
L.C.C.H., Morley College, 61 Westminster Bridge Road, London  SE1 7HT
*Disabled Access*
L.C.C.H. Homoeopathic Clinic, telephone for appointment: 071-928 6199

---

## THE GENERAL COUNCIL AND REGISTER OF
## CONSULTANT HERBALISTS

WITH

## THE REGISTER OF HOMOEOPATHIC PRACTITIONERS

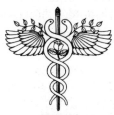

OFFER:

Full curriculum of training in Herbal Medicine and/or Homoeopathic Practice leading to membership as a Registered Medical Herbalist (M.R.H.) and/or Registered Homoeopathic Practitioner (D.Ho.M.). Training is carried out initially by correspondence courses, followed by practical clinical training.

New syllabus available from February 1992. For further details send large stamped addressed envelope to:

The Secretary, G.C.R.C.H., Grosvenor House, 40 Sea Way, Middleton-on-Sea, West Sussex  PO22 7SA. Tel: 0243 586012

# The Scottish College of Homœopathy

Principal:Margaret Roy B.A.hons.

PROFESSIONAL TRAINING IN HOMŒOPATHIC MEDICINE
4 year FULL-TIME COURSE (Advanced)
4 year FULL-TIME COURSE (Ordinary)

STARTS OCTOBER 1991
The objective of the College since its inception in 1985 is to train Homœopaths to practice Classical Homœopathy to the highest standard. To achieve this the College course places a strong emphasis in clinical training and on medical sciences. Each section of the course is intergrated with the others and teaching takes place in small groups in carefully graduated stages.

CORRESPONDENCE COURSES
Principles & Practice of Homœopathy
Homœopathic Materia Medica

Originally set up to cater for the rural student in the Highlands and Islands these are not professional courses in themselves but it is possible to use the course to gain exemption from the First Year of College professional course. Summer School and examinations are then compulsory.

For more details and an application form write to

The Secretary,
The Scottish College of Homœopathy,
17 Queens Crescent, Glasgow, G4 9BL.

# THE COLLEGE OF CLASSICAL HOMOEOPATHY

## 4 YEAR PART-TIME PROFESSIONAL TRAINING COURSE
From September to June

&

## SUPERVISED CLINICAL TRAINING
For the complete 12 months in the latter stages.

Apply to:
The Registrar
45 Barrington Street,Tiverton, Devon  EX16 6QP
Tel: 0884 258143

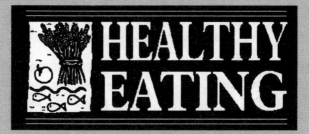

## No Other Magazine Concentrates On Healthy Eating As Much As We Do

Now we're more concentrated than ever with an issue

# Every Month

Where matters of food are concerned
*HEALTHY EATING*
is concerned about Food Matters

Make certain that you keep right up to date on the
very latest by buying
*HEALTHY EATING* Magazine

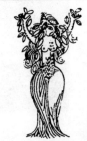

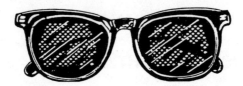

# Waterless Cookware

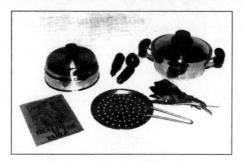

## SPECIALLY DESIGNED
## FOR A HEALTHIER WAY OF COOKING

This superb cooking system utilises an improved method of cooking and suits most cookers.

* COOKING WITHOUT WATER to retain the natural nutrients in food.

* COOKING WITHOUT UNNECESSARY FAT to minimise the dangers of a high-fat diet and to alleviate or prevent conditions such as high blood pressure, cholesterol, heart disease, obesity, digestive problems etc.

* Food which retains natural mineral salts requires less flavouring, salt and fatty sauces.

### Ordinary food suddenly acquires more taste!

WATERLESS COOKWARE is a complete system of cooking which has revolutionised the kitchen. Made of CR/NI-18/10 Stainless Steel with a SPECIAL THERMIC BASE the utensils can boil, roast, fry, bake, braise, grill etc. and can be used on the table. Environmentally friendly in the kitchen it is safe, easy to clean, hygienic, energy saving and leaves the kitchen and work tops clean and without odours and condensation.

### Unlimited Guarantee

An UNLIMITED GUARANTEE MAKES WATERLESS COOKWARE excellent value for money.

WATERLESS COOKWARE is for health..... not just for cooking.

Available exclusively from:-

BRITIMCO WATERLESS COOKWARE (U.K.)
Brendon House
Langham Road
Robertsbridge
East Sussex  TN32 5DT
Tel: (0580) 880262

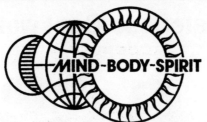

# Festival for Mind-Body-Spirit

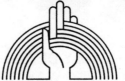

## Healing Arts Exhibition

*organised by*
New Life Designs
Arnica House
170 Campden Hill Road, London W8 7AS
Tel: 071-938 3788  Fax: 071-723 7256

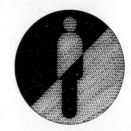

# Appendix 3

# RECOMMENDED READING

*The Biochemic Handbook.*
J. S. Goodwin, paperback, £2.50

*The Complete Homoeopathy Handbook.*
Miranda Castro, 257pp, paperback, £12.99

*Homoeopathic Medicine:*
*A Doctor's Guide to Remedies for Common Ailments.*
Trevor Smith, 256pp, paperback, £6.99

*The Magic of the Minimum Dose.*
Dr. Dorothy Shepherd, 216 pp, hardback, £8.95

*The Organon of Medicine.*
Samuel Hahnemann, 270pp, paperback, £9.99

*The Science of Homoeopathy.*
George Vithoulkas, 154pp, paperback, £9.99

*Vaccination and Immunisation:*
*Dangers, Delusions and Alternatives.*
Leon Chaitow, 156 pp, paperback, £6.99

All page extents and prices are subject to change (both up and down!) without notification from the publishers.

The above listed books are available from:
Hyden House Ltd., Little Hyden Lane, Clanfield, Hampshire PO8 0RU
Telephone 0705 596500 Fax 0705 595834

*Please add £1 per book towards postage and packing.*
*For orders of 4 books and over add £3 towards postage and packing.*

Hyden House also supply books on a wide variety of other subjects from Permaculture and environmental issues to helping your child learn to read. Please ask for our *Holistic Emporium* catalogue.

# Index

chronic prescribing 7-9
civilised diseases 1
colds 73-4
colic 90, 95
comfrey 50
   ointment 38
common sense 50, 151
complementary medicine 35
concussion 141
confidence
   lack of 52-4, 56
conjunctivitis 65-7
constipation 97-8
contraceptive pill 6-7, 107
coughs 80-2
counselling 35, 37
cramps
   muscular 116
   stomach 86
cystitis 99-100

dandruff 122
DDT 6
decimal scale 23
depression 51-9
despondency 55-7
diarrhoea 95-6
diphtheria 13
diuretics 6
dosage 45-6
double blind trials 19
drug dependent culture 5-7
drug picture 18, 19, 21, 45
dysentery 1

ears
   boils 68
   catarrh 68-9
   earache 68-9
   discharges 68-9
   Hopi ear candles 68
   wax 68
emotional problems 30, 51-9
empowerment 3, 40
Euphrasia 65
exercise 31
eyes
   black 141

conjunctivitis 65-7
   discharges 65-7
   impaired vision 65-7
   photophobia 65-7
   styes 65-7

fear 52-4, 58
   of operations 143
fevers
   chicken pox 123-4
   colds 73-4
   ear 68-9
   German measles 125-6
   glandular fever 127-8
   influenza 129-30
   measles 131-2
   mumps 133-4
   throat 77-7
   tonsillitis 135-6
first aid 139-45
   course 8, 139
   prescribing 44-5
food 27-9
fractures 142

Gaia 39-40
German measles 125-6
glandular fever 127-8
golf 31
Graphites 39
grief 56, 58

haemorrhoids 93
Hahnemann, Samuel 10, 11-7, 25, 49
hair
   loss of 122
hayfever 75-6
headaches 61-4
heart
   congenital malformations 9
   coronaries 7
   disease 1, 28, 30
heartburn 85-7
hepatitis 1
Herring, Constantine xvi, 46
Hippocrates 12, 37
holistic vision 27